Marc-Olivier Sauvain

Studies on lentiviral-mediated transgenesis

Marc-Olivier Sauvain

Studies on lentiviral-mediated transgenesis

Südwestdeutscher Verlag für Hochschulschriften

Impressum/Imprint (nur für Deutschland/ only for Germany)

Bibliografische Information der Deutschen Nationalbibliothek: Die Deutsche Nationalbibliothek verzeichnet diese Publikation in der Deutschen Nationalbibliografie; detaillierte bibliografische Daten sind im Internet über http://dnb.d-nb.de abrufbar.

Alle in diesem Buch genannten Marken und Produktnamen unterliegen warenzeichen-, marken- oder patentrechtlichem Schutz bzw. sind Warenzeichen oder eingetragene Warenzeichen der jeweiligen Inhaber. Die Wiedergabe von Marken, Produktnamen, Gebrauchsnamen, Handelsnamen, Warenbezeichnungen u.s.w. in diesem Werk berechtigt auch ohne besondere Kennzeichnung nicht zu der Annahme, dass solche Namen im Sinne der Warenzeichen- und Markenschutzgesetzgebung als frei zu betrachten wären und daher von jedermann benutzt werden dürften.

Verlag: Südwestdeutscher Verlag für Hochschulschriften Aktiengesellschaft & Co. KG
Dudweiler Landstr. 99, 66123 Saarbrücken, Deutschland
Telefon +49 681 37 20 271-1, Telefax +49 681 37 20 271-0, Email: info@svh-verlag.de
Zugl.: Lausanne, ETH, Diss, 2009

Herstellung in Deutschland:
Schaltungsdienst Lange o.H.G., Zehrensdorfer Str. 11, D-12277 Berlin
Books on Demand GmbH, Gutenbergring 53, D-22848 Norderstedt
Reha GmbH, Dudweiler Landstr. 99, D- 66123 Saarbrücken
ISBN: 978-3-8381-0579-6

Imprint (only for USA, GB)

Bibliographic information published by the Deutsche Nationalbibliothek: The Deutsche Nationalbibliothek lists this publication in the Deutsche Nationalbibliografie; detailed bibliographic data are available in the Internet at http://dnb.d-nb.de.

Any brand names and product names mentioned in this book are subject to trademark, brand or patent protection and are trademarks or registered trademarks of their respective holders. The use of brand names, product names, common names, trade names, product descriptions etc. even without
a particular marking in this works is in no way to be construed to mean that such names may be regarded as unrestricted in respect of trademark and brand protection legislation and could thus be used by anyone.

Publisher:
Südwestdeutscher Verlag für Hochschulschriften Aktiengesellschaft & Co. KG
Dudweiler Landstr. 99, 66123 Saarbrücken, Germany
Phone +49 681 37 20 271-1, Fax +49 681 37 20 271-0, Email: info@svh-verlag.de

Copyright © 2008 Südwestdeutscher Verlag für Hochschulschriften Aktiengesellschaft & Co. KG and licensors
All rights reserved. Saarbrücken 2008

Produced in USA and UK by:
Lightning Source Inc., 1246 Heil Quaker Blvd., La Vergne, TN 37086, USA
Lightning Source UK Ltd., Chapter House, Pitfield, Kiln Farm, Milton Keynes, MK11 3LW, GB
BookSurge, 7290 B. Investment Drive, North Charleston, SC 29418, USA
ISBN: 978-3-8381-0579-6

Contents

Chapter 1   Introduction

1.1 The lentivirus..1
1.2 The lentiviral vector..2
    1.2.1 Controlling gene expression from and with lentiviral vectors................6
    1.2.2 Genomic integration of retroviruses..10
1.3 Animal transgenesis..12
    1.3.1 Lentiviral vector-mediated transgenesis...14
    1.3.2 Lentiviral vector: broadening the perspectives of transgenesis...........16
        1.3.2.a Large transgenic animals...16
        1.3.2.b Transgenic knockdown animals..17
        1.3.2.c Conditional transgenesis and knockdown..................................18
        1.3.2.d Generating transgenic animals from ES cells...........................18
1.4 Early steps of mammalian development..20
1.5 Gene expression in early pre-implantation embryos....................................22
1.6 Studying mammalian genetics through mutagenesis...................................24
    1.6.1 Generalities...24
    1.6.2 Gene trap vectors..26

Chapter 2   Genotypic features of lentiviral-derived transgenic mice

2.1 Introduction..28
2.2 Material and methods..29
    2.2.1 Lentiviral-mediated transgenesis..29
    2.2.2 LAM PCR..30
    2.2.3 Cloning, sequencing, and annotation of LAM PCR products.............31
    2.2.4 ISS PCR..32
    2.2.5 RNA expression measurements..32
2.3 Published study...34
2.4 Conclusion..44
    2.4.1 Lentiviral integration: a retrospective analysis..................................45
    2.4.2 Integration site analysis..51
    2.4.3 Limitations of lentiviral-mediated transgenesis.................................55
    2.4.4 LAM and integration sites..56

Chapter 3   Study of lineage commitment of early blastomere

3.1 Introduction..58
3.2 Material and methods..60
    3.2.1 Lentiviral-mediated transgenesis...60
    3.2.2 Southern blot...60
3.3 Results..61
    3.3.1 Lentivectors to analyse blastomeric fate...61
3.4 Conclusion...63
    3.4.1 Benefits and limitations..65
    3.4.2 The prepatterning vs. regulative model...69

Chapter 4   Development of a new lentiviral gene trap vector

4.1 Introduction..70
4.2 Material and methods..71
    4.2.1 Lentiviral trap vector...71
    4.2.2 ES cells culture...72
    4.2.3 LacZ staining...73
4.3 Results and discussion...73
    4.3.1 Overview..73
    4.3.2 Experimental perspectives for a lentiviral gene trap vector.............77

Bibliography..81

Addendum 98

Chapter 1
Introduction

1.1. Lentivirus:

Lentiviruses belong to the Retroviridae, a large and diverse family of enveloped RNA viruses defined by common taxonomic denominators that include structure, composition and replicative properties[9]. The hallmark of the Retroviridae family is its replicative strategy, which includes the reverse transcription of the virion RNA into linear double stranded DNA and its subsequent genomic integration. All retroviruses contain three major coding domains with information for virion proteins: gag, which directs the synthesis of internal virion proteins that form the matrix, the capsid, and the nucleoprotein structures; pol, which contains the information for the reverse transcriptase, integrase and protease enzymes; and env, from which the surface and transmembrane components of the viral envelope protein are derived. Simple retroviruses usually carry only this essential information, whereas complex retroviruses code for additional regulatory non-structural proteins derived from multi-spliced messages.

The Retroviridae family can be further subdivided into Orthovirinae and Spumavirinae. The Orthovirinae sub-family is further divided into 5 different generi, amongst which the lentiviruses (Fig. 1). The prefix lenti- derives from the latin word "lentus" meaning slow and is related to the slow progression of the diseases caused by these viruses, ranging from interstitial pneumonia in sheep (Visna/Maedi virus) to the acquired immuno-deficiency syndrome (Human immuno-deficiency virus, HIV), a disease that has killed more than 30 million individuals in some thirty years of pandemics.

Chapter 1. Introduction

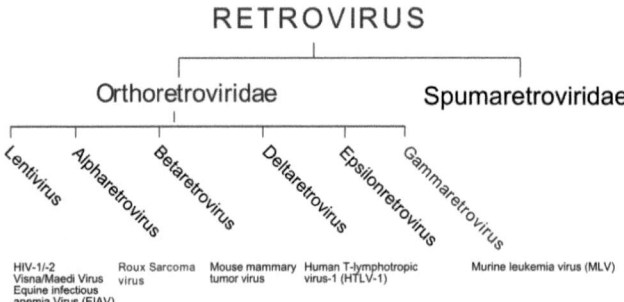

Fig. 1. Schematic representation of the retroviridae family. Representative members of selected generi are indicated.

1.2 Lentiviral vectors:

The development of viral vectors should be placed in the context of technologies that emerged during the late seventies and early eighties to introduce foreign genes into mammalian genomes[10-15]. The Herpes virus thymidine kinase gene was the first sequence to be exogenously delivered by calcium-phosphate mediated transfection into mammalian cells[16, 17]. Among the different techniques that were subsequently generated, virus-based vectors became an attractive tool to increase the efficiency of gene transfer and to broaden its application to in vivo settings[18]. The prototypic Moloney murine leukaemia virus (MLV) became a battle horse for such experiments as it has a relatively large capacity (around 7kb of foreign material), a wide host range, long terminal repeats providing efficient signal for initiation and termination of transcription, and most importantly because it integrates its cargo into target genomes[19-22]. However, one major drawback of MLV is its inability to infect non-dividing cells, such as cardiomyocytes, neurones or stem cells[23, 24]. Interestingly, lentiviruses can infect both dividing and non-dividing cells[25]. The original demonstration that an HIV-based vector could mediate stable gene delivery in vivo into non-dividing cells came with the injection of lentiviral vector into the central nervous system of rats[26]. The integrated proviruses were able to provide a strong and long lasting expression of the transgene into neuronal cells. This was due to their ability to hijack the cell nuclear import machinery and to cross the nuclear envelope in an energy-dependent manner[27, 28]. The determinants of this property were mapped to specific viral components: the matrix (MA), virion protein R (Vpr) and integrase (IN)[29-32]. The tropism of HIV-derived vectors was broadened owing to the use of envelopes derived from other viruses, such as the G protein of the vesicular stomatitis virus (VSV-G). This envelope is also advantageous due to its high stability, allowing the concentration of high-titer vector stocks by ultracentrifugation [33, 34]. Furthermore, early in the development of lentiviral vectors, major efforts were devoted to increase their biosafety[35].

In addition to containing the prototypic gag, pol and env genes common to all retroviruses, lentiviruses encode two regulatory proteins, Tat and Rev, both essential for replication, as well as several accessory factors playing important roles in pathogenesis. However, not all these elements are crucial for the making of a lentiviral vector, allowing for a great gain in biosafety. All four accessory genes (vif, nef, vpu and vpr) can indeed be deleted without affecting gene transfer efficiency[35]. Tat, the potent transactivator that plays a pivotal role in HIV replication, can be removed as well. Its role during HIV infection ranges from the trans-activation of the full length viral RNA to the expression of different cellular genes such as TNF alpha and beta and IL-2[36]. The trans-acting function of Tat is dispensable if another transcriptional unit replaces the viral promoter. Enhancer elements from the Rous sarcoma virus promoter regions or from the immediate-early promoter of CMV were found to substitute efficiently for Tat-dependent sequences in the 5' LTR.

Self-inactivating (SIN) lentiviral vectors, obtained through the almost complete deletion of the U3 region of the HIV 3' LTR in the plasmids used to generate the vector genome, add to the biosafety of the system[37, 38]. The U3 region contains the retrovirus essential transcriptional elements such as enhancers and promoter. Therefore, U3-deleted vectors result in transcriptionally deficient LTRs in the resulting provirus, further decreasing the risk of replication-competent recombinant viruses (Fig 2). This design also diminishes the potential impact of viral endogenous sequences on the transcriptional activity of cellular coding sequences located adjacent to the integration site, as well as possible interference between the LTR and the exogenous promoter used to express the transgene.

Altogether, the conservation of only three (gag, pol and rev) out of the nine genes contained in the HIV genome and the SIN design of the packaged vector reduce the risk of generation of replication-competent recombinants to close to null, thus allowing for a broad use of lentiviral vectors for basic research and clinical applications alike.

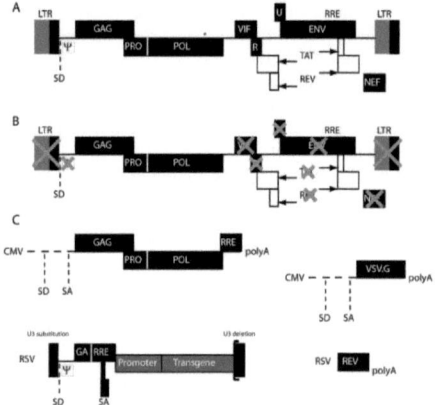

Fig. 2. From HIV-1 to a lentiviral vector. A. Schematic drawing of the wild type HIV provirus. B. The different deletions leading to the production of the third-generation HIV1-derived packaging construct. C. The 4-plasmid system required to produce the third-generation lentiviral vector: the split gag-pol/rev packaging constructs, the heterologous envelope (in this case VSV-G) plasmid and the SIN transfer vector. (Adapted from Lentiviral Vectors, Ed. D. Trono, 2002, Springer-Verlag)

Chapter 1. Introduction

Currently, the production of the so-called third generation lentiviral vector is achieved by transient transfection of four different plasmids in producer cells[39]. The gag and pol genes encoding for structural and enzymatic proteins are on the same plasmid. The env gene, generally that encoding the G protein of vesicular stomatitis virus, is on a second plasmid. A third plasmid contains the rev gene and a fourth plasmid the sequence coding for the vector itself, that is, the only RNA that will be transferred into target cells. While this so-called third-generation system is favoured for clinical use, a simpler second-generation version (in which gag, pol and rev are on the same plasmid) is preferred for laboratory studies (Fig. 2). Thus, the routine production of lentiviral vector is based on the transient transfection of only three plasmids into a so-called producer cell, most often the 293T cell line derived from human embryonic kidney cells. The following day, the cells are washed with fresh medium. Within the next 48 hours, the vectors will accumulate in the supernatant, which will be collected so as to yield, after ultracentrifugation, the concentrated vector stock. Usual titres are in the range of 1×10^8 to 1×10^9 HeLa transducing unit/ml (Fig. 3).

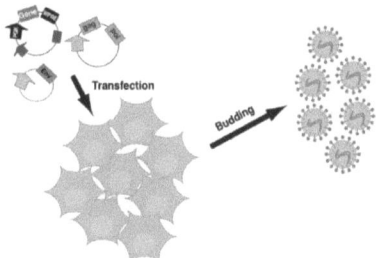

Fig. 3. Schematic drawing of a typical second-generation lentiviral vector production. Three plasmids are co-transfected in permissive cells (usually 293T cells): the packaging construct, the heterologous envelope plasmid and the transfer vector DNA. During the following 48h, viral particles will be produced and secreted into the supernatant. A careful collection of this supernatant and its ultracentrifugation will lead to a high-titer viral preparation.

1.2.1 Controlling gene expression from and with lentiviral vectors

Since its early development in the late nineties, the lentiviral vector system has been improved in two major aspects: biosafety and control of transgene expression[40].

One priority following stable integration of a provirus is the correct expression of its DNA cargo independently of the surrounding genetic environment. Therefore, solutions to isolate transcriptionally the integrated virus (the provirus) from the surrounding took advantage of sequences called insulators. Early work done on insulators was carried out in D. melanogaster using the gipsy retrotransposon[41]. The insertion of this element within enhancer-rich regions was found to block effectively the action of all enhancers that were distal to its site of integration. The proposed mechanism involves numerous cellular genes leading to the formation of DNA clusters- insulators bodies- localized at the nuclear periphery[42]. In vertebrates, the first insulator found lied within the 5' end of the chicken beta-globin locus[43, 44]. This complex element called cHS4 exerts its anti-enhancer activity through the binding of CCCTC-binding factor (CTCF), an evolutionary conserved and ubiquitously expressed vertebrate zinc finger protein[45-47]. One important role of CTCF is the regulation of the imprinted gene insulin-growth factor 2 (Igf2). In embryonic tissues, Ifg2 is expressed only from the paternal allele and under the control of downstream enhancers. Between Igf2 and these enhancers lies a so-called imprinted control region (ICR) containing multiple binding sites for CTCF. Paternal-specific methylation of theses sites preclude the binding of CTCF and its anti-enhancer activity allowing Igf2 activation from the downstream enhancer-regions[48, 49]. The molecular basis of CTCF insulator activity is not completely elucidated but mostly relies on its ability to form clusters with other CTCF molecules generating closed loop domains[50]. Another interesting strategy to prevent the surrounding genetic landscape from influencing the expression of the transgene uses an "enhancer trap decoy". This system consists of a strong promoter immediately followed by transcription terminators. The idea is that this construction placed upstream of an expression cassette will soak transcriptional activity coming from the surrounding host genome and stop it at its terminator element. This kind of construction was successfully used to analyze the periodic activity of circadian genes[51]. Preventing potential "genetic interference" from host DNA on transgene expression is an important issue when the latter has to be restricted to a given cell type in vivo. A contrario, the host DNA should be protected from cis-acting influences coming from an integrated retrovirus nearby or to potential detrimental effects of the transgene in non-target cells. One possibility to avoid diffuse expression of the transgene is to use tissue-specific promoters. Numerous tissue-specific promoters exist covering a vast range of cell types[52-54]. Another way is to control exogenously the expression of the proviral DNA. One of the best characterized systems to achieve such an effect is based on the Tet operon and repressor, and was successfully implemented into the lentiviral vector platform[55, 56]. This method enables the transient expression of genes by controlling their transcription upon administration of the antibiotic tetracycline or one of its derivatives. Basically, a fusion protein -the tetracycline transactivator protein (tTA) - composed of the Escherichia Coli Tetracycline repressor and the viral protein 16 of Herpes simplex virus, a potent and ubiquitous transactivator, binds to the tetracycline operator (tetO) sequence upstream of a minimal CMV promoter. Upon binding of the tTA to the tetO operator sequence, VP16 strongly stimulates the transcription of the downstream gene. This interaction can be modulated by the administration of tetracycline, which displaces the tTA from its target DNA, thus shutting down transcription. This system is therefore called the Tet-off system. A Tet-on counterpart was further developed taking advantage of a mutant Tet repressor that requires tetracycline for specific DNA binding[57]. Both systems were successfully applied to the lentiviral backbone to control transgene expression in various organs such as the central nervous or the hematopoietic systems[58, 59]. Thus by coupling a Tet system to a tissue-specific promoter, a precise activation in time and space can be achieved[60]. The discovery that mammalian gene expression could be controlled post- transcriptionally using small interfering RNAs (siRNAs) opened new perspectives to investigate gene function by reverse genetics[61, 62]. In organisms or cells with weak or no interferon responses to double stranded RNA, constructs that express long hairpin under a Pol II promoter can be used, allowing inducible, tissue- or cell-type specific RNA expression[63]. In order for the siRNA to be used in mammalians cells without triggering the apoptotic cascade, expression systems using a Pol III promoter were developed[64, 65]. Briefly, this polymerase triggers the production of small hairpin RNAs (shRNAs) that are further processed by an RNase III enzyme complex (DICER) into functional siRNA duplexes. Then, an endonuclease complex uses these siRNAs as a guide to cleave the homologous mRNA sequence resulting in a decrease in steady-state of the targeted mRNA[66, 67]. The incorporation of shRNA into lentiviral vectors was achieved by placing a shRNA sequence into the 3' LTR downstream of a pol III promoter such as H1 or U6[68]. The interest of this design is multiple. First, upon retrotranscription the Pol III-shRNA cassette will end up duplicated in both LTRs. Second, the expression cassette driven by a Pol II promoter is still developed with various degrees of success[69]. In our laboratory, we took advantage of epigenetic regulators to control siRNA expression[70]. The tetracycline repressor was fused to the Krüppel associated box domain (KRAB). KRAB-containing DNA binding proteins inactivates transcription through the formation of heterochromatin within a few kilobases (kb) upstream and downstream of its binding site precluding access to DNA for transcription factors, whether recruited within the context of pol II or pol III promoters. A TetO was cloned upstream of the shRNA expression cassette and used thereby as a docking site on which tTR-KRAB could repress transcription in a tetracycline-controllable manner (Fig. 4). This expression system was used successfully in vitro and in vivo to down-regulate conditionally various genes[70, 71]. Recently, the discovery that mammalian cells synthesize microRNAs (miRNAs) to control endogenous genes at a post-transcriptional level gave new insights into RNA interference. Hundreds of these miRNAs are encoded by the human genome, and are believed to play key roles in vertebrate differentiation and development[72]. MiRNAs are transcribed by type II polymerase as pre-miRNAs precursors. A first interaction with an RNase III enzyme (Drosha) produces an approx 65nt pre-miRNA. This precursor is then extruded into the cytoplasm where a second RNase III enzyme (DICER), a common pathway with the siRNA, will cleave it to its active form consisting of approx 25 nucleotides. This RNA interacts with RISC components and together they can trigger the down regulation of homologous mRNA. New lentiviral developments are taking advantage of the Pol II dependence of the miRNA to control in a regulated (either tissue-specific or drug-controlled) manner the expression of endogenous genes[73].

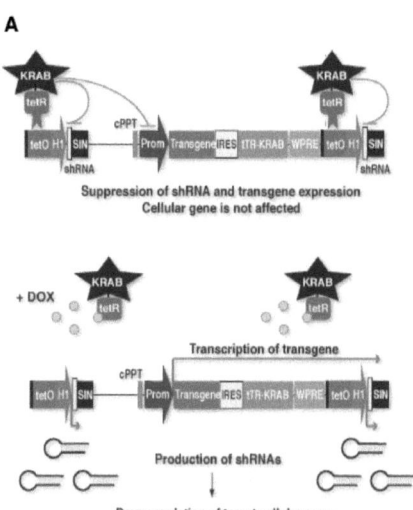

Fig.4. Schematic representation of a lentivirus containing the TET-on system. Upon administration of doxycycline, the Tet-KRAB fusion protein is removed from its docking site (TetO) and allows the transcription of the shRNA, leading to the downregulation of the target cellular gene. When doxycycline is removed the Tet-KRAB fusion protein interacts again with the tetO site and stops the transcription by inducing epigenetic modifications. Abbr: SIN: self-inactivating LTR, IRES: internal ribosomal entry site, WPRE: woodchuck post-regulatory element, KRAB: Krüppel-associated protein. (Adapted from Szulc et al, Nat Methods. 2006 Feb; 3(2): 109-16.)

1.2.2 Genomic integration of retroviruses

The improvement of retroviral vectors within the past few years opened new hopes for the treatment of clinical conditions such as monogenic congenital disorders, for which standard therapies are often disappointing[40]. Such diseases include cystic fibrosis, certain forms of immunodeficiency, Criggler-Najar syndrome, familial phenylalaninemia and many others[74-77]. The idea is to bring exogenously a gene into an organism presenting a defective version of it. The first unambiguous success for human gene therapy was reported in 2000 when children presenting a severe form of X-linked immunodeficiency were successfully treated using retroviral vectors carrying the missing genetic information[78]. During the first round of clinical experimentation 10 young patients were treated. However, the first serious adverse effects occurred in 4 patients, who developed a leukemia-like lymphoproliferative disease[79, 80]. Interestingly, in the two adverse events reported in details to date, integration of the therapeutic vectors, a gammaretrovirus-derived vector, occurred upstream of the same proto-oncogene LMO2, leading to its activation and ultimately to leukaemia[81, 82]. Unfortunately, 1 patient died from this complication, while the three others could be saved following appropriate chemotherapy and bone marrow transplant. This serious complication stimulated efforts to characterize the genomic features of retroviral integration[83]. Mitchell et al analyzed 3127 integration sites of three retroviral vectors derived from MLV, HIV-1 and avian sarcoma-leukosis virus (ASLV) in cell lines and primary cells[84]. Interestingly, these three vectors showed discrete modes of integration site selection. MLV exhibited a strong integration bias near transcriptional start sites[84], while HIV favoured the transcribed region of genes. While these two delivery systems targeted preferentially active genes, ASLV showed no bias for these, nor for promoter regions (Fig.5).

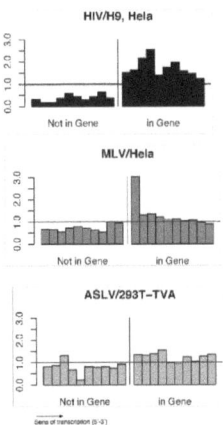

Fig. 5. Integration frequency in genes and intergenic regions. Genes or intergenic regions were normalized to a common length and then divided into ten intervals to allow comparison. The number of integration sites in each interval was divided by the number of matched random control sites and the value plotted. A value of one indicates no difference between the experimental sites and the random controls. Viruses and cell types studied are as marked above each graph. (Adapted from Mitchell et al, PLoS Biology Vol. 2, No. 8.)

The molecular mechanisms underlying integration site selection are still not clearly understood. However, a study showed that replacement of the HIV integrase by that of MLV influenced the integration site selection of HIV[85]. Namely, this hybrid HIV vector-MLV integrase tended to target integration near transcriptional start sites and CpG island-rich regions, recapitulating the integration preferences of MLV. The addition of MLV gag within this construction further increased the similarity of target site selection to that of MLV. This finding suggests that the integrase plays a pivotal role in the selection of integration site, probably through its tethering to host proteins bound near preferred genomic regions. Recently, the LEDGF/p75 cellular factor was identified as a potential tethering factor implicated in HIV integration[86]. A simple model holds that one domain of LEDGF/p75 binds to the HIV preintegration complex and another binds chromatin near active transcriptional units. In this model, LEDGF/p75 should accumulate near active transcriptional units, although this has not been demonstrated to date. Moreover, it is not known whether LEDGF/p75 recognizes alone active regions or is guided via histone post-translational modifications, as suggested by one study[87]. Within the past few years, lentivector-mediated transgenesis has emerged as an alternative to pronuclear injection to generate transgenic mice[88]. A detailed discussion of the pattern of proviral integration in mice generated by this technique will be provided in the following chapters.

1.3. Animal transgenesis

All animal species are, sensu largo, transgenic, as during evolution they all have incorporated into their genome various forms of foreign DNA, especially of viral origin. However, the term transgenic is used in a more restrictive fashion to designate animals that have some foreign DNA integrated in their germ line as a consequence of experimental procedures[2, 89]. According to this definition, the first attempt to generate transgenic animals was conducted more than thirty years ago by the in vitro injection of SV40 viral DNA into the cavity of blastocysts, an early stage of the developing mouse embryo composed of a few hundred cells[90]. The embryos were introduced into the uterus of a surrogate mother and allowed to develop to term. The viral DNA integrated at very low frequency the genome of some of the most superficial cells surrounding the cavity, generating mosaic animals carrying only a few transgenic cells in their tissue. Nevertheless, these pioneer experiments proved that exogenous DNA could stably integrate the genome of an embryo without impinging on its future development. However, due to the very limited number of transgenic cells, the transmission of the transgene from one founder to its offspring was never observed, hindering the use of this method to generate lines of transgenic animals. In an effort to increase the amount of transgenic cells within the embryo, and thus to increase the probability of germ-line transmission, viruses replaced naked DNA. The prototypic Moloney murine leukaemia virus (MLV) was chosen as it was known to introduce its own genome into the host chromosomes[91]. Moreover, as this virus was able to make its way from the cell surface to the nucleus, the need to visualize or to manipulate morphological structures such as the blastocoel cavity was not a prerequisite, allowing therefore the use of embryos at earlier stages of development. MLV particles were incubated overnight with day 2-3 embryos, which were then transferred to surrogate mothers. Interestingly, a few pups not only developed leukaemia, thereby proving the incorporation of the viral sequences into their genome, but some of them were also able to transmit leukaemia to the next generation[92]. This experiment stimulated scientist to develop recombinant MLV containing genes with potential therapeutic application[93, 94]. However, these subsequent experiments were frustrating as the expression of transgenes was poor or inexistent within the offspring[95]. This phenomenon was attributed to the de novo hypermethylation of the viral LTRs known to contain CpG dinucleotides, resulting in silencing.

Nevertheless, these seminal studies stimulated the scientific community to discover other methods to bring exogenous DNA into host genome while preserving the expression of the transgene. One of the techniques developed took advantage of cell culture to first introduce transgenes into teratocarcinoma cells line and subsequently to transfer the nucleus of these cells into the cytoplasm of an enucleated embryo[96]. Although this technically challenging technique brought some success, it raised questions about its use as the transferred nuclei were plagued with genetic instabilities.

A breakthrough came in the early 80th when Gordon et al described the use of mechanical injection of plasmid DNA directly into one of the pronuclei of a fertilized oocyte[97]. The mechanical pressure applied during the microinjection on the pronucleus breaks randomly the host chromatin at different points, allowing exogenous DNAs to find their way between broken chromatins and stably incorporate the host genome following DNA repair. The first DNA injected was a plasmid containing a fragment of simian SV40 virus containing the coding sequence of the thymidine kinase gene (TK) of Herpes simplex virus. Out of 19 mice obtained using this technique, 3 presented sequences homologous of the injected plasmid out of which one exhibited TK activity in the liver and the kidney[98]. Within a couple of years, the pronuclear injection of naked DNA became the new standard to generate transgenic animals. However, this technique, as the others, still carries a low efficiency rate

Chapter 1. Introduction

considering that only 3% of the microinjected embryos generate transgenic animals. This number increases to about 20% when counting living mice only. That is, in a normal pregnancy containing around 10 pups, 2 are transgenic[3]. However, this number should be corrected for the percentage of transgenic animal correctly expressing the transgene, roughly 50% of cases - although some specific transgenes are expressed in higher proportions- and that only transgenic male are-for obvious reasons-conserved[99].
Pronuclear injection has also been used to modify genetically other species than mus musculus[3]. Thus, transgenic farm animals, including pigs, rabbits and sheep were successfully generated. However, for those animals the efficiency of transgenesis is so low (less than 1%) that the cost of production can reach up to 300'000 US dollars for a transgenic cow, which precludes the use of pronuclear injection as a routine technique to generate transgenic livestock[100]. The difficulty to visualize the pronuclei of these species from the surrounding opaque cytoplasm accounts in part for this low efficiency. But as discussed later, a new technique taking advantage of the lentivirus greatly simplifies the generation of transgenic livestock.

1.3.1 Lentiviral vector-mediated transgenesis

Although pronuclear injection is still the method of choice to generate transgenic animals, the fact that it is relatively inefficient, technically demanding, costly and mostly impracticable in other species than mouse prompted the development of other techniques. Ideally, any new technology had to be simple to perform, efficient in term of number of animals expressing correctly the transgene, and applicable to multiple species. The previous use of retroviruses as a tool to generate transgenic mice raised the possibility that lentiviral vectors might be advantageous. The risk of epigenetic silencing during early development, as reported for MLV, seemed reduced since most of the HIV cis-acting sequences within the LTR were deleted in common lentiviral vectors[40]. The proof-of-principle was brought in 2002 with the lentivector-mediated generation of transgenic mice and rats[101]. In this experiment, a vector carrying a GFP reporter gene driven by a ubiquitous promoter was injected between the plasma membrane of fertilized oocytes and its glycoproteinic outer membrane, called the zona pellucida. The space between these two membranes is called the perivitelline space and can be clearly visualized next to the polar body where the zona pellucida loops out.

Chapter 1. Introduction

Once into this perivitelline space, the vector anchors to the plasma membrane, penetrates into the cytoplasm by receptor-mediated endocytosis and finally integrates into the chromosomal DNA. The results obtained were encouraging as more than 30% of injected embryos produced transgenic animals, as compared to 3% using pronuclear injection. Moreover, these transgenic animals expressed the transgene in more than 80% of the case. Interestingly, the approach was successfully applied to the rat, a species known to be difficult to manipulate genetically. This experiment produced transgenic rats at a frequency of 59% using the same lentiviral construction, with a rate of transgene expression as high as 40%. These figures are to be compared with the 17,4% efficiency of rat transgenesis using pronuclear injection. Finally, expression of GFP could be restricted to a given tissue using tissue specific promoters such as those of myogenin, active in skeletal muscles, or lck, active in T cells only.

Lentivirus-mediated transgenesis (LVT) was not only superior to pronuclear injection to generate transgenic animals from different species than mus musculus but drastically reduced the technical skills required for such operation (Fig.6). In order to simplify further the procedure, lentiviral vectors were co-incubated for a few hours with embryos, the zona pellucida of which had been previously removed by acidic treatment. Embryos were then extensively washed and transferred to surrogate mothers, following thereafter the same procedures as for LVT. The efficiency of the procedure drops significantly but the percentage of transgenic animal is comparable to that obtained by the pronuclear injection[102].

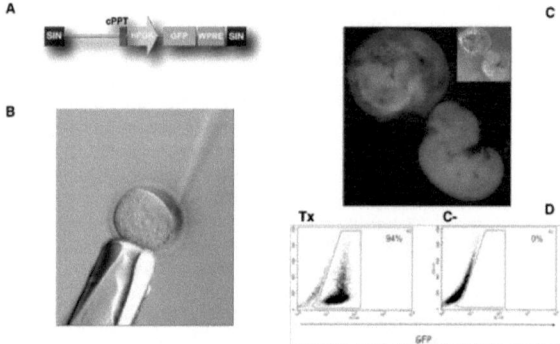

Fig. 6. Lentiviral-mediated transgenesis. A. Schematic drawing of the vector used in this experiment containing a ubiquitous promoter, the human phosphoglycerate kinase promoter, and GFP as reporter gene B. Perivitelline injection of a methylene blue solution. C. Fluorescent microscopy showing a transgenic embryo with its placenta. Bright field image also depicted.
D. FACS analysis from the peripheral blood from a different animal containing a similar lentiviral construct. This analysis shows a uniform expression of eGFP. (Tx. Transgenic animal. C-: negative Control).

1.3.2 Lentiviral vector: broadening the perspectives of transgenesis

1.3.2.a. Large transgenic animals

Transgenic technologies have emerged as invaluable tools to manipulate the genome of multiple organisms in biomedical, veterinary and agricultural research[3]. Techniques at hands are multiple, but today the method of choice to generate transgenic mammals remains the pronuclear injection of naked DNA into fertilized oocytes. Unfortunately, this approach is hampered by a relatively low efficiency, particularly in species other than mice. The urge to overcome this limitation is pressing, owing to the importance of species such as pigs, goat, sheep, rabbits and many others for studying biological functions and for developing new medical treatments. Although the inefficiency of pronuclear injection can be overcome in small animals such as mice by playing the numbers, that is, by generating a large progeny and screening for pups with proper transgene integration, this is an unpractical endeavour in larger species such as sheep, goat or cows, be it only because of its extreme costs. Lentiviral vectors offer the opportunity to fill this niche, owing to their ease of delivery into early embryos from numerous species [103]. Studies performed in cows and pigs have shown very high levels (93-100%) of transgene integration following lentivector-mediated transduction of oocytes. The rate of transgene expression in the founders was also encouraging, as it reached 64% in pigs and 100% in cows[103].

1.3.2.b. Transgenic knockdown animals

Transgenic approaches have largely involved the overexpression of various transgenes, but the advent of RNAi in mammals allowed the production of transgenic animals with the ability to decrease the expression of endogenous genes[104]. As discussed previously, an interesting feature brought by the lentiviral vector technology is its ability to down-regulate the expression of endogenous genes via RNA interference. Upon infection of embryos with shRNA-carrying lentiviral vectors, all cells within the transgenic animal should contain RNAi sequences. In a study, shRNA targeted against GFP in double transgenic (GFP+/GFPshRNA+) mice significantly reduced GFP expression in the founders and progeny F1 mice[105]. However, the demonstration that an endogenous gene could be efficiently down-regulated came from a study using shRNA against CD8 T cell surface marker[106]. Transgenic mice overexpressing CD8 shRNA silenced CD8 expression up to 90% in developing thymocytes, compared to control mice. However, the loss in the number of mature CD8+ cells (20-100%) did not directly correlate with the decreased level of gene expression. Interestingly, another study observed that the silencing of Slc11a1, which downregulates the Nramp1 protein, reduced the incidence of diabetes mellitus in non obese diabetic (NOD) mice, following genetic modification of their zygote with lentiviral vectors carrying Slc11a1 shRNA. Of note, the NOD mouse is a strain that is notoriously difficult to manipulate using standard pronuclear injection[107].

1.3.2.c. Conditional transgenesis and knockdown

The down-regulation of a gene can have unwanted side effects if exerted ubiquitously or can impinge on development leading ultimately to embryonic death. The Cre-Lox system was one of the first choices for controllable shRNA expression in transgenic animals as it was already widely used to regulate gene expression in this field[108]. This system originates from the loxP-Cre site-specific recombination system present on the intact P1 bacteriophage plasmid[55]. The recombinase Cre catalyzes reciprocal recombination at a specific locus of crossing over (lox). The lox sequence is composed of two 13-base-pair (bp) inverted repeats separated by an 8-bp spacer region. Upon binding to the inverted repeats, Cre synapses with a second lox site and then cleaves the DNA in the spacer region to initiate strand exchange with the synapsed lox partner. No additional factors are required for the recombination and this action is not reversible. Thus, the transcription of shRNA can be locked by a spacer, containing or not coding sequences, introduced between the TATAA box of a Pol III promoter and the beginning of the shRNA. As this spacer is flanked with two LoxP sites, the Cre enzyme, upon activation, can excise this spacer and put the Pol III promoter back in a suitable configuration to trigger transcription of the downstream shRNA. As many mouse strains express Cre in specific organs, they can be crossed with transgenic animals carrying a "locked" shRNA, producing thereafter within the offspring shRNAs activation in tissues where Cre is transcribed. An "off-system" was also developed where LoxP sites flanked the shRNA-expressing cassette. Upon Cre activation, the whole cassette is removed, allowing the targeted RNA to be expressed again. A new inducible version of the Cre-Lox system offers the flexibility to activate the expression of CRE upon administration of tamoxifen[109].

1.3.2.d. Generating transgenic animals from ES cells

Embryonic stem cells are derived from early mammalian embryos and display characteristics of totipotency, i.e., after transfer to a suitable in vivo environment they can contribute to the primary germ layers (ectoderm, endoderm, and mesoderm) and populate the germline of mice[110]. The success of the lentiviral vector in transgenesis prompted its use to generate transgenic animal derived from transduced ES cells. Although ES cells are partially

Chapter 1. Introduction

resistant to lentiviral transduction in vitro, high doses of vector overcome this limitation. An interesting feature while working with ES cells is the in vitro screening phase before their introduction within the cavity of a blastocyst. This blastocyst carrying two genetically distinct populations of cells will create a chimeric animal made of exogenous ES cells as well as endogenous blastocyst cells. The degree of chimerism is reflected by the coat colour of the animal, if exogenous ES cells and the resident blastocyst code for different colours.

However, the long time needed to get a progeny from a chimeric founder, due to the relatively poor germ-line transmission of ES cells, prompted the development of a new procedure that could bypass this step. A high electric field can fuse the plasmatic membrane of 2 cell-stage blastomeres leading to the generation of a tetraploid genome[111]. These blastomeres develop until the blastocyst stage but are unable to sustain further the embryonic development. However, the injection of 2n ES cells within the blastocoele cavity of a tetraploid embryo will rescue the developmental failure of these tetraploid cells and generate an animal derived exclusively from the ES cells. Interestingly, under these conditions, the tetraploid cells are still able to contribute to the extra-embryonic development. Therefore, complementation of tetraploid blastomeres with normal ES cells results in the production of embryos entirely derived from the injected ES cells. Thus, the time between the first cloning of the vectors to the transgenic mouse can be reduced to the minimum[112]. However, only hybrid ES cells lines can sustain the development of tetraploid embryos, probably because of the hybrid vigour[113].

Thus, Ventura et al transduced ES cells with lentiviral vectors containing shRNA against CD8, locked by a spacer containing a strong promoter and a GFP as reporter gene, creating thereby the first transgenic animal derived from transduced ES cells[114]. They selected 3 GFP+ clones and transferred ES cells into the cavity of a tetraploid blastocyst. Out of the 3 transgenic founders, 2 of them produced a GFP+ progeny. To achieve either a global or a tissue-specific activation of shRNA-that is the removal of the spacer cassette following Cre activation- the authors crossed this progeny with MSX2-Cre or Lck-Cre respectively. Both strains showed a specific reduction in splenic CD8+ but not CD4+ T lymphocytes as compared with controls. As expected, the shRNA CD8+/MSX2-Cre double transgenic mice showed a complete excision of the spacer cassette, lacking thereby any GFP+ expression, whereas shRNA CD8+/Lck-Cre mice presented GFP- cells in the thymus only. As stated in this study, tetraploid blastocyst complementation could generate conditional knockdown mice in as fast as 5-6 weeks following manufacture of the lentiviral constructions.

1.4. Early steps of mammalian development

During the first few days of life, the embryo establishes its polarity building from the original one-cell symmetry a dorso-ventral, right-left and head-tail asymmetry that will determine the body plan of the whole animal. In various organisms such as C. elegans, Drosophila melanogaster or Xenopus laevi, the plan of polarization is already embedded within the cytoplasm of the one-cell stage embryo[115-117]. This is achieved by the programmed distribution during gametogenesis and subsequent fertilization of morphogenetic determinants within discrete zones of the cytoplasm. In Drosophila, for example, oogenesis builds morphogenic differences within the oocyte[118, 119]. Thus, the polar distribution of the bicoid mRNAs coding for a homeodomain-containing transcriptional factor modulates the patterning of the embryo[120]. The translation of bicoid mRNA triggered by fertilization eventually creates a morphogenic gradient that patterns the anterior region of the embryo through the transcriptional activation of the gap and pair rule genes along the anterior-posterior axis. Interestingly, transplantation of cytoplasm taken from this region can induce the formation of anterior structures at ectopic sites. Thus, the early mammalian development was long believed to be an exception to the rule that the embryo polarity takes its root from the spatial patterning of the egg[4, 121]. The embryo was considered as a blank sheet till the late blastocyst stage as experimental manipulations of early blastomeres did not end in gross developmental abnormalities, whereas in other organisms it would have disrupted early patterning[122, 123]. Thus, blastomeres issued from 8 cells stage embryos could be used to generate twins or triplet, providing that their early development is supported by tetraploid cells (4n)[124]. Moreover the body axes of the embryo become apparent only at the end of the first week of development corresponding to one third of the whole gestation in mouse. This first sketch of body axes appears at a significantly later stage of development in mammals than other animals. The importance of gastrulation for the mammals was quoted by the biologist Lewis Wolpert:" It is not birth, marriage, or death, but gastrulation, which is truly the most important time in our life"[6]. To date, no molecules have been identified within the mammalian

Chapter 1. Introduction

embryo that could mimic the effects of morphogenetic determinants, such as the bicoid in Drosophila. These morphogenetic considerations lead to the conclusion that mammalian development should be highly regulative, meaning that cell fates were allocated dynamically and relatively late through cell-cell interactions and that this process was not due to an uneven distribution of morphogenetic cues among individual blastomeres[121]. Interestingly, some embryologists consider the blastocyst stage in mammals as the equivalent of the one cell stage in non-mammals based on their functional properties (Hiiragi, personal communication). However, recent studies suggest that even if cellular fate is not determined from the zygote on, a bias could exist as early as the two-cell stage[8, 125-127]. As no molecules were discovered that could be linked to a specific cell fate, this assessment is based on morphological cues. That is, on the establishment of correlations between early cleavage plans and subsequent cell fate, through lineage tracing experiments. Such studies showed that the first two cleavages of the fertilized oocyte were predictive of the embryonic and abembryonic axis of the blastocyst in 80% of the analyzed embryos. To determine if these four blastomeres, issued from the first two cleavages, had different regulatory properties, these cells were dissociated and mixed according to their spatial position[126]. Cells near the second polar body represented the animal pole and the others the vegetal pole. Interestingly, embryos induced from blastomeres originating exclusively from the vegetal pole failed to develop to term, while blastomeres issued from the animal poles resulted in a normal progeny, suggesting that these vegetal and animal poles blastomeres, though morphologically identical, already present different intrinsic properties. In the present work, we showed that during early development the progeny of the first blastomeres tend to be diversely represented among embryonic and extraembryonic tissues, suggesting an early bias in their cell fate.

1.5 Gene expression in early pre-implantation embryos

During the first days of life, an embryo will have to cope with radical reprogramming of its genome. Different waves of transient de novo transcription will govern the preimplantation development[128]. This embryonic period encompasses the formation of the zygote with the fusion of the two pronuclei to its implantation into the uterine wall about 4.5 days after conception. The first major genomic alterations come along with the generation of haploid oocytes and spermatozoids. Female gametogenesis starts during foetal life with a massive proliferation of germ cells and a blockade by birth at the diplotene stage of the first meiotic division. During reproductive life, oocytes are continuously selected to grow from the pool of small primordial oocytes reaching full size in 2 weeks. During this time, the cellular machinery will establish a maternal store of materials to support fertilization and preimplantation development. At the time of ovulation, the oocyte will have completed the first meiotic division and will be blocked at the metaphase of the second meiotic division. (H3) uridine incorporation studies showed a marked decrease in transcription at that stage[129]. The translational activity remained but at very low level. Thus, from the fertilization to the first division, the metabolism of the embryo will mostly rely on maternally derived transcripts and proteins[130]. This transcriptional quiescence necessitates post-transcriptional and post-translational mechanisms to orchestrate the multitude of processes participating in meiotic maturation, fertilization, and reprogramming of the nascent embryonic genome. However, 90% of maternal mRNA will be degraded at the two cells stage, suggesting that the time window for embryonic genomic activation is very narrow[131]. In fact, a minor transcriptional activity already occurs in the male pronucleus 5 hours post-fertilization, followed by the female one, at a lower level, as shown by brUTP incorporation studies[132]. This minor activation is linked to DNA replication suggesting that the degradation of the nucleosomes give access for the maternally derived transcription machinery to promoters that were previously not accessible. However, this minor activation is weak and results in the synthesis of a small set of polypeptides that transiently increase at the two cells stage[133]. Following the first division, the ensuing major zygotic genome activation (ZGA) entails a dramatic genomic reprogramming ending by the complete switch of genetic control from maternally derived transcripts/proteins to the newly formed embryonic genome[131, 134, 135]. No longer than one division later at the 4 cells stage, another major genomic activation, called mid-preimplantation gene activation (MGA), takes place preparing the morphological changes that first begin from the 8-cells stage on. The last activation during the preimplantation period is observed between the morula and the blastocyst stage, but less than 100 genes are activated de novo[128].

The mechanisms and molecular pathways underlying genome reprogramming and the start of a new life remain poorly understood, largely because the functional analyses of single genes and pathways dominate in this field of developmental biology. However, alternative approaches, such as large-scale transcriptome analysis, emerge as a useful "reverse genetics" tool for extraction of essential information. For instance, one study followed the different stages of early embryonic genome activation at a transcriptome level using a microarray composed of ca. 22000 genetic features[128]. Five pools of 500 embryos each representing the important embryonic stages were probed against it. In silico analysis identified 9 clusters of ca 12000 statistically significant genes that were further assigned to 3 main groups. Schematically, the first group represented genes that were newly activated from the zygotic genome. The second group contained genes abundant in the oocytes decreasing during the preimplantation period and the third group combines features of group one and two (that is transiently activated from the zygotic genome). Group two and three are of particular interest because they contain clusters of genes showing a transient de novo transcription within a narrow time window. This means that some of these genes will drive the different waves of zygotic activations during their brief activation and then shut off. For example, 82% of the 4216 genes activated for the first time during the MGA fall into 1 clusters of the third group. This cluster of genes shows a transient increase from the 4 to 8 cells stage followed by a rapid decrease from the 8 cells stage to morula. Moreover, the list of genes activated from MGA on includes many known genes important for ES cells homeostasis such as Nanog, Pou5f1 or Lefty1 and other more implicated in trophoblast stem cells, such as Gata3 or endoA. Thus, early embryonic development is governed on one hand by wave of transient gene activation resetting the genetic environment and on the other hand by a regulated constitutive activation of gene that will build the future embryo. Interestingly, the generation of the totipotent zygote is driven by maternally derived transcripts/proteins stored during the maturation of the oocyte.

1.6 Studying mammalian genetics through mutagenesis

1.6.1 Generalities

With the sequencing of many genomes now completed, tools are at hands to determine the physiological role of every single gene. Reverse genetics, whereby phenotypes of interest are first identified and then assigned to specific genotypes, is a powerful means to reach at least partly this goal. However, since the frequency of naturally occurring mutations in a given gene is extremely low (5×10^{-6} per locus) and since such mutations range from hardly detectable single nucleotide changes to chromosomal rearrangements, various strategies were developed to induce mutations more efficiently. X-ray mutagenesis was the first technique used for its tendency to produce mutations of a relatively defined molecular nature at a frequency about 20-100 times greater than spontaneously occurring mutations[136]. As X-rays trigger chromosomal rearrangements, they produce readily detectable landmarks. However, these chromosomal alterations involve most of the time many genes, making the results difficult to interpret. Therefore, agents that can introduce mutations into single genes are favoured. Ethylnitrosourea (ENU) is an alkylating agent that is a powerful mutagen in mouse spermatogonial stem cells, producing single locus mutations at a frequency of 6×10^{-3} to 1.5×10^{-3}, equivalent to obtaining a mutation in a single gene of choice in one out of every 175 to 655 gametes screened[137-139]. The analysis of germline mutations reveals that ENU predominantly modifies A-T base pairs, mostly A-T to T-A transversions and A-T to G-C transitions. When translated into a protein product, the diverse changes result in missense mutations, nonsense mutations, and splicing errors. The ratio loss-of-function versus gain-of-function mutations is 1:4[139]. Moreover, ENU is easy to administer and can introduce many different mutations in a single male that can then be mated for many months to generate a highly diverse mutant progeny. However, as ENU produces point mutations, the search for a given phenotype-causing genotypic alteration is costly and time-consuming as it requires out crossing breeding strategies, SNP sequencing, and positional cloning[140]. Nevertheless, ENU driven mutation was successfully used as critical start point to characterize important genes and pathways such as the clock gene involved in circadian rhythm[141].

Chapter 1. Introduction

In stark contrast to the hit-and-miss character of these strategies is the programmed nature targeted mutagenesis by homologous recombination in ES cells[142-144]. Since its first use to disrupt the hypoxanthinephosphoribosyl transferase gene, gene targeting was intensively used to study gene function and structure[145, 146]. Sequences homologous to host target gene are usually encompassing a cassette containing a gene to be inserted (LacZ, eGFP, antibiotic resistance...). These homologous arms will find their way to their cellular counterparts and appose closely to them. Rarely, this will trigger the cell homologous recombination machinery to introduce the cassette within desired locus, disrupting the architecture of the recipient gene. However recombination events in mammalians cells occur at a very low frequency ranging from about 1 out of 100 treated cells. Therefore a positive selection cassette is mandatory to retrieve the positive ES cells. As one major limitation remains the high frequency of random (non homologous) integrations, a negative selection cassette is also contained within the targeting construct but outside the homology arms, so that it will be incorporated into the host genome only when a non-homologous recombination happened, which occurs in mammalian cells in about 1 cell out of 100 treated cells. Following a positive and negative selection, ES cells are used to make chimeric animals[147]. Subsequent breeding will generate transgenic animals carrying the mutagenized locus on both alleles. As potent as this technique may be, numerous KO mice lack any obvious characteristics. This lack of phenotype can reflect the compensatory effect of parallel pathways. Such a scenario could explain why a KO can present a wide variation of phenotype ranging from not detectable to early death depending on the mouse strain used. In such cases, strain differences reflect the importance of the genetic background in which the disrupted gene resides.

Gene trapping takes the middle path between random and molecularly defined mutations[148-150]. The introduction of gene-trap vectors into the mouse germ line through ES cells has permitted random mutations to be generated and characterized in vitro before germ-line transmission. Gene trap vector can be electroporated as DNA plasmid or incorporated within a viral vector to infect the target cells. Both methods can be scaled-up to perform high-throughput analyses. Thus, large gene trap screens were built in order to saturate the entire ES cells genome with insertions. In 2004, nearly two third of the calculated 30'000 mouse genes were trapped by these multicentric studies and ES cells clones are now publicly available (www.genetrap.org). However, the rate of newly trapped genes is decreasing presumably reflecting the integration site preferences of any single vector. Thus, the diversification of the type of gene trap vector seems to be a prerequisite to saturate completely the mouse genome.

1.6.2 Gene trap vectors

A prototypic gene trap vector contains a splice acceptor (SA), a strong polyA signal that is located downstream of a reporter cassette but lacks a promoter. Thus, gene trap vectors are unable to drive the expression of their transgene and need to be integrated within introns, where they hijack the transcriptional machinery at their own use and stop it prematurely at their polyA signal. Splicing will then occur between the splice donor site (SD) of the incomplete endogenous transcript and the SA of the gene trap. This chimeric sequence will be further processed into a fusion protein containing the reporter (Fig.7). Although the original activity of the protein will be either null or partial, the expression of the reporter gene, often consisting of a fusion between a LacZ and an antibiotic resistance cDNA, allows for the positive selection of ES cells having incorporated the gene trap vector within active genes. To circumvent the loss of inactive trapped genes, a resistance cassette lacking polyA signal is inserted into the gene trap vector downstream of a constitutive promoter. This resistance marker is then expressed only if the vector integrates into a gene, active or not, to benefit from its polyA signal. Following positive selection, the sequence of the gene trap vector will be used as a tag to recover the site of integration. As gene trap vector rely entirely on endogenous cis–acting promoter and enhancer elements, they show a pattern of expression reflecting that of the targeted endogenous genes. Thus, the in-vivo expression of the targeted gene can be monitored when a transgenic mouse is generated. Moreover, as gene traps usually disrupt the function of the trapped gene, the homozygous state will lead to a null mutation producing an overt phenotype in 60% of the cases according to one study[151].

Chapter 1. Introduction

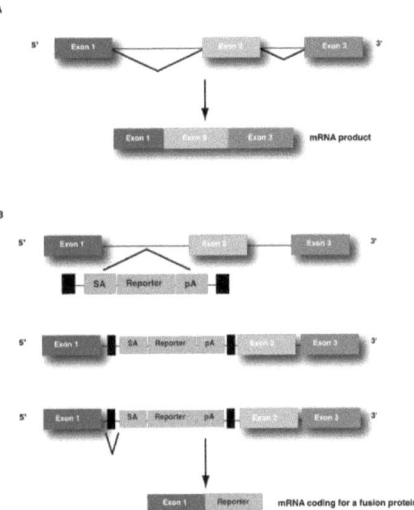

Fig. 7. Gene trap mechanism. A. Normal transcription unit producing an endogenous mRNA. B. Integration of a gene trap into the same locus. The gene trap will be transcribed along with the endogenous gene up to the exogenous polyA signal. Then, this transcript will hijack the endogenous processing of mRNA to achieve a fusion protein containing both part of the endogenous sequence and the gene trap sequence.

Chapter 2
Genotypic features of lentiviral-derived transgenic mice

2.1 Introduction

Within the past 5 years, lentiviral vectors have emerged as an attractive tool to generate transgenic animals[101]. While conventional micro-injection based methods for transgenesis were successful in producing small and large transgenic animals, they are still hampered by a relatively low efficiency and high costs, particularly in species other than mice[99, 152]. This is a considerable challenge to overcome because of the importance of species such as pigs, goat, sheep, rabbits and many others for studying biological function and developing new biomedical treatment in humans[3]. Although the inefficiency of pronuclear injection transgenesis can be overcome in small animals by high-throughput screening for DNA integration, this type of approach becomes economically more challenging in larger animals[103]. For this reason, new strategies to enhance the production and the variety of transgenic animals would be valuable and an important asset to the scientific community. One emerging technique has been the use of lentiviral vectors as an alternative tool for transgenesis as they are effective gene transfer vehicles that mediate a stable integration of their DNA cargo into a vast repertoire of cell types from a wide variety of species[101]. In a typical procedure, the lentiviral vector is injected into the perivitelline space underneath the zona pellucida of the zygote. After fusion with the plasma membrane, its viral RNA penetrates into the cytoplasm and undergoes reverse transcription yielding a double stranded DNA that eventually integrates the host chromosome[101]. Both, the time required by the lentiviral vector to get into the cellular DNA and the time needed by the zygote to divide will define the degree of genotypic mosaicism found in the resulting animal. Integration events occurring subsequent to the first cell division will limit the presence of individual proviruses to at most 50% of the cell population of the embryo. The phenotypic consequences of this mosaicism can usually be minimized through the use of vector doses high enough to induce multiple proviral copies per embryo, ensuring that all cells harbour at least one integrant. However, the degree of genotypic mosaicism of the founder (G0) animal conditions the rate of transmission of individual proviruses to its (G1) progeny. In the present study, we investigated the degree of genetic mosaicism associated with lentiviral transgenesis in mice and found that it is minimal, suggesting that viruses integrate rapidly when injected into the mouse zygote.

Furthermore, the integrated provirus could influence the host genetic regulation by exerting cis-acting effects, a phenomenon known as insertional mutagenesis. The best-characterized example of this phenomenon comes from the first successful gene therapy clinical trial performed on SCID children using MLV-based vectors. In four out of 14 children treated to date, MLV cis-activated proto-oncogenes in the vicinity of their integration site, leading to the development of acute leukaemia. Large-scale analysis in vitro of retroviral integration sites revealed that vectors derived from MLV or HIV tend to favour active genes but in different manner. Whereas MLV tends to integrate in and around promoter regions, HIV targets transcribed regions. Here, we performed an in vivo analysis of HIV integration sites within transgenic mice generated by the lentiviral infection of preimplantation embryos.

2.2 Material and methods

2.2.1 Lentiviral-mediated transgenesis

We generated transgenic mice by perivitelline injection of fertilized oocytes, as described [101]. Briefly, the hybrid strain B6D2G1 derived from C57BL/6JxDBA2J (Charles River, France) was used as egg donor. Superovulation was induced by intra-peritoneal (IP) injection of five B6D2G1 female with 10 IU of Pregnant Mare Serum (PMS) (Sigma, Buchs, Switzerland). Forty-six hours later, a second IP injection was performed with 10 IU of Human Chorionic Gonadotropin (HCG) (Sigma), before mating with B6D2G1 males. Sixteen hours later, oocytes were harvested, injected in the perivitelline space with a highly concentrated vector stock (5×10^8-1×10^9 HeLa transducing unit/ml), and kept in culture overnight at 37°C and 5% CO_2 in KSOM medium (Specialty Media). Embryos that had reached the 2-cells stage were then placed in the ampulla of foster NMRI mothers (8 embryos per ampulla). All vectors used in this study were previously described [70]. Genotyping of the offspring was done by PCR using vector-specific primers (forward primer: 5'-TATGTTGCTCCTTTTACGCTATGTG-3, reverse primer: 5'-CGACAACACCACGGAATTGT-3').

2.2.2 LAM PCR

DNA of transgenic mice was purified by standard phenol/chloroform extraction and ethanol precipitation and DNA of NIH3T3 fibroblasts grown in DMEM 10% FCS (Invitrogen, Paisley, UK) was purified with the DNeasy extraction kit according to the manufacturer's recommendation (Qiagen, Hilden, Germany). Linear-amplification mediated (LAM)-PCR was carried out as described [153] with minor modifications. 5 ng genomic DNA was mixed in a 50 µL reaction with 1x Taq DNA polymerase buffer (Qiagen), 200 µM dNTPs (Sigma, Buchs, Switzerland), 2.5 nM oligo AD30 and AD31 (all primers are listed in supplementary Table 3) and 2.5U Taq polymerase (Qiagen). Primers were extended after initial denaturation for 5' at 94°C (hot start) followed by 50 cycles of 94°C for 1', 60°C for 45", 72' for 1'30 and a final extension at 72°C for 10'. Dynal kilobasebinder beads (Invitrogen) were washed 2x with 0.1% BSA in PBS and resuspended in 50µL of binding buffer provided with the kit and added to the PCR at final concentration of 20 µL beads per PCR. Extension products were captured for 1h at room temperature under agitation and washed with water. 2nd strands were synthesized in 20 µL reactions containing 1x hexanucleotide buffer (Roche, Rotkreuz, Switzerland), 30 µM dNTPs, and 2 U Klenow (Roche) for 1h at 37°C. Beads were washed with water and digested in 20 µL containing 4 U of Tsp509I (New England Biolabs, Allschwil, Switzerland) and 1x buffer #2 for 1h at 65°C. Beads were washed with water and ligated in a 10 µL reaction containing 1x Fast-Link buffer (Epicentre, Dottikon, Switzerland), 1 mM ATP, 2 µL of AD25/AD26 linker cassette and 2 U Fast-Link ligase for 5' at room temperature. Beads were washed with water and denatured for 10' at room temperature with 5 µL 0.1 M NaOH. 2 µL of this LAM-product was exponentially amplified in 50 µL reactions containing 1x Taq DNA polymerase buffer (Qiagen), 200 µM dNTPs (Sigma), 500 nM oligo AD27 and AD32 and 5 U Taq polymerase (Qiagen). Primers were extended after initial denaturation for 3' at 94°C (hot start) followed by 35 cycles of 94°C for 45", 60°C for 45", 72' for 45" and a final extension at 72°C for 10'. 1 µL of this PCR product was amplified in a 50 µL reaction with 1x Taq DNA polymerase buffer (Qiagen), 200 µM dNTPs (Sigma), 500 nM oligo AD33, 400 nM AD28, 100 nM AD62 and 5 U Taq polymerase (Qiagen). 1 µL of the final PCR product was mixed with 0.5 µL Rox GeneScan standard (Applied Biosystems, Switzerland) and 8.5 µL distilled formamide (Applied) and denatured for 2' at 95°C. PCR reactions were separated on a 3100 sequencer (Applied) and analyzed with the GeneScan software.

2.2.3 Cloning, sequencing, and annotation of LAM PCR products

PCR reactions were purified with a Nucleobond II kit (Macherey-Nagel, Switzerland) and eluted in 30 µL 5 mM TRIS-HCl pH 8.0. 15 µL of this eluate was digested overnight with 5 U NarI (NEB) in a 20 µL reaction at 37°C. 0:6 µL of this digest was mixed in 96-well plates with 0.5 µL pCR4-TOPO (Invitrogen) and 0.4 µL salt solution in a final volume of 2.3 µL. After incubation for 5' at room temperature, reactions were heat-shocked into DH5alpha provided with the kit (Invitrogen). Colonies were picked into 96-well plates and sequenced at GATC Biotech, Konstanz, Germany. Sequences were extracted from chromatograms using phred [154]. Vector and HIV contaminating sequences plus U5 and LC fragments were identified with blast [155], and removed prior to annotation. Mouse repeats in the cleaned sequences were identified and masked with RepeatMasker. The location of each cleaned, masked sequence in the mouse genome (NCBIm34 assembly) was determined with megablast [156] using a word length of 24. The annotation procedure was automated using a series of ad hoc perl scripts. Gene-relative mappings were determined using the ENSEMBL database (http://oct2006.archive.ensembl.org/). We defined genes as transcription units annotated in the ENSEMBL database; data tables were assembled in

OpenOffice 2.0 and statistical analysis performed with R or PRISM 4.0 software.

2.2.4 ISS PCR

Site specific PCRs were exponentially amplified in 25 µL reactions containing 100ng of DNA, 1.5x Taq Polymerase buffer (Qiagen), 200 µM dNTPs (Promega), 0.8 µg BSA (NEB), 25 mmol MgCl2 (Qiagen), 5 U of hotstart Taq polymerase (Qiagen) and 200 nM. The PCR reaction started with an initial activation step of 95°C for 15 min (Hotstart), followed by 10 cycles of 94°C 45'', 60°C (-1°C per cycle) for 45'', 72°C for 1' (touchdown), and 30 cycles of 94°C for 45'', 50°C for 45'', 72°C for 1' and a final extension at 72°C for 10'. 5 µl of loading buffer (6x) were added to each PCR reaction and 15 µl were run on a 0.8% agarose gel for about 30' at 80V before analysis under UV

2.2.5 RNA expression measurements

NIH3T3 fibroblasts were cultured in DMEM/10% FCS (Invitrogen) at 37°C and 5% CO_2 and Oct4-GiP (kind gift A. Smith, Edinburgh, UK) ES cells were cultured as described [157] in the presence of 500 ng puromycin (Sigma)/mL at 37°C and 10% CO_2. RNA was isolated with TRIZOL (Invitrogen) and ethanol precipitation according to standard procedures and cDNA synthesized with hexanucleotides according to manufacturer's recommendation using the SuperScript III first strand cDNA synthesis system (Invitrogen). 50 unfertilized eggs or 2-cells embryos were resuspended in 1 µL RNAse out and 10 µL resuspension buffer (SuperScript III CellsDirect cDNA synthesis system; Invitrogen) and denatured for 10' at 75°C. DNase digestion was carried out according the manufacturer's instructions and 2 µL of 50 ng/µL hexamers added with 1 µL dNTPs. Reactions were denatured at 70°C for 5' and remaining reagents added as indicated in the protocol. Reactions were left for 10' at 25°C before reverse transcription. RNase H digested cDNAs were used for quantitative PCR The expression of each gene was assayed in triplicate in a total volume of 5 µl containing 1x POWER SYBR (Applied Biosystems), 200 nM each gene-specific primer pair (see table), and diluted cDNA (cultured cells 1:17 and embryonic cDNA 1:2.6). To verify specificity, each PCR was followed by a melting-curve analysis and minus RT samples were run in parallel. The increase in fluorescence was analyzed with SDS 2.2.2 software (Applied Biosystems). For all amplification plots, the baseline data were set with the automatic CT function available with SDS 2.2.2, calculating the optimal baseline range and threshold values by using the AutoCt algorithm (SDS 2.2 user's manual). A mean quantity was calculated from triplicate PCR reactions for each sample, and this quantity was normalized to two similarly measured quantities of normalization genes as described [158]. Normalized quantities were averaged for three replicates for each data point and represented as the mean±s.d. The highest normalized relative quantity was arbitrarily given a value of 1.0. Fold changes were calculated from the quotient of means of these normalized quantities and reported as ±s.d.

Chapter 2. Genotypic features of lentiviral-derived transgenic mice

2.3 Published study

Genotypic Features of Lentivirus Transgenic Mice[▽][†]

Marc-Olivier Sauvain,[1] Alexander P. Dorr,[1][‡] Brian Stevenson,[2] Alexandra Quazzola,[1] Félix Naef,[1] Maciej Wiznerowicz,[1] Frédéric Schütz,[2] Victor Jongeneel,[2] Denis Duboule,[1,3] François Spitz,[3][§] and Didier Trono[1]*

School of Life Sciences and Frontiers in Genetics National Center for Competence in Research, Ecole Polytechnique Fédérale de Lausanne, Lausanne, Switzerland[1]; Ludwig Institute for Cancer Research and Swiss Institute of Bioinformatics, 1015 Lausanne, Switzerland[2]; and Department of Zoology and Animal Biology, University of Geneva, Geneva, Switzerland[3]

Received 20 March 2008/Accepted 30 April 2008

Lentivector-mediated transgenesis is increasingly used, whether for basic studies as an alternative to pronuclear injection of naked DNA or to test candidate gene therapy vectors. In an effort to characterize the genetic features of this approach, we first measured the frequency of germ line transmission of individual proviruses established by infection of fertilized mouse oocytes. Seventy integrants from 11 founder (G0) mice were passed to 111 first generation (G1) pups, for a total of 255 events corresponding to an average rate of transmission of 44%. This implies that integration had most often occurred at the one- or two-cell stage and that the degree of genotypic mosaicism in G0 mice obtained through this approach is generally minimal. Transmission analysis of eight individual proviruses in 13 G2 mice obtained by a G0-G1 cross revealed only 8% of proviral homozygosity, significantly below the 25% expected from purely Mendelian transmission, suggesting counter-selection due to interference with the functions of targeted loci. Mapping of 239 proviral integration sites in 49 founder animals revealed that about 60% resided within annotated genes, with a marked tendency for clustering in the middle of the transcribed region, and that integration was not influenced by the transcriptional orientation. Transcript levels of a set of arbitrarily chosen target genes were significantly higher in two-cell embryos than in embryonic stem cells or adult somatic cells, suggesting that, as previously noted in other settings, lentiviral vectors integrate preferentially into regions of the genome that are transcriptionally active or poised for activation.

Transgenic animals are essential research tools, whether they are used to address basic biological questions or to develop preclinical models of human diseases. Their generation through the injection of naked plasmid DNA into the male pronucleus of fertilized oocytes has been a standard practice for almost 3 decades (5), but the success of this procedure has been largely limited to mice. Recently, lentiviral vector-mediated transgenesis has emerged as an attractive alternative, as these human immunodeficiency virus (HIV)-derived gene transfer vehicles can mediate the efficient integration of their cargo into zygotes or early progenitors from a wide variety of species including mice, rats, pigs, cows, and chickens (4, 8, 13, 20, 23). In a typical procedure, the lentivirus particle is injected beneath the zona pellucida of a fertilized oocyte and penetrates this cell by fusion between the viral and plasma membranes. Its RNA genome then undergoes reverse transcription, yielding a double-stranded DNA copy that integrates into the host cell chromosomes.

The kinetics of lentivirus integration into the target genome defines the degree of genotypic mosaicism found in the resulting animal. Integration events occurring subsequent to the first cell division will, indeed, limit the presence of individual proviruses to only a subset of cells and, hence, condition their rate of transmission to the first generation (G1) progeny. Even though the phenotypic consequences of this mosaicism can usually be minimized through the use of vector doses high enough to induce multiple proviral copies per embryo, ensuring that all cells harbor at least one integrant, individual proviruses are subjected to different influences conditioned by their site of integration into the host genome (8). Furthermore, the integration site of individual proviruses will influence their potential to exert cis-acting effects on the host genome, a process known as insertional mutagenesis. Large-scale analyses of retroviral integration sites in somatic cells have revealed that, while vectors derived from both murine leukemia virus (MLV) and HIV favor active genes, the former tend to integrate in and around promoters, whereas the latter rather target transcribed regions (14, 19, 30). Noteworthy, when MLV vectors are used to infect early mouse embryos, they are rapidly silenced during development, in contrast to their lentiviral counterparts (9). It is not known whether this partly reflects differences in integration site selection or results solely from the sequence-specific recruitment of epigenetic repressors, such as recently demonstrated for the primer binding site-dependent KAP1/TRIM28-mediated silencing of MLV vectors in embryonic stem cells (28, 29).

The present work presents a genotypic characterization of transgenic mice obtained from oocytes injected with lentiviral vectors. It demonstrates that integration occurs rapidly follow-

* Corresponding author. Mailing address: Ecole Polytechnique Fédérale de Lausanne, School of Life Sciences, Station 15, Lausanne CH-1015, Switzerland. Phone: 41 21 693 1751. Fax: 41 21 693 1635. E-mail: didier .trono@epfl.ch.
‡ Present address: Merck Serono International S.A., 9 Chemin des Mines, 1202 Geneva, Switzerland.
§ Present address: EMBL, Meyerhofstr. 1, 69117 Heidelberg, Germany.
† Supplemental material for this article may be found at http://jvi .asm.org/.
▽ Published ahead of print on 7 May 2008.

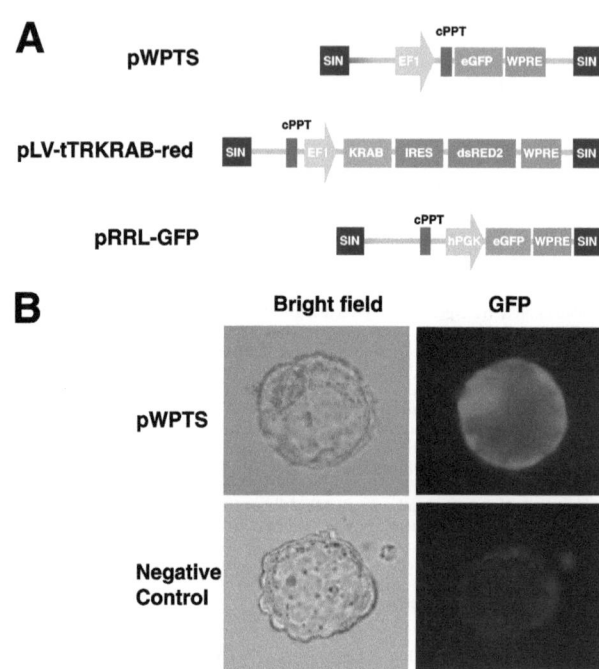

FIG. 1. Lentivirus transgene expression in blastocysts. (A) Schematic representation of lentiviral vectors used in this study. Abbreviations: SIN, self-inactivating LTR; WPRE, woodchuck hepatitis posttranscriptional regulatory element; IRES, internal ribosomal entry site; cPPT, central polypurine tract; hPGK, human phosphoglycerate promoter; CAG, chicken actin-globin chimeric promoter; KRAB, tetracycline repressor-KRAB fusion protein. (B) Transduction of fertilized oocytes after perivitelline injection of pWPTS vector. eGFP expression is detected in the trophectoderm and the inner cell mass of the blastocyst (top); a blastocyst derived from an uninfected oocyte is shown as a control (bottom).

ing this procedure, so that the degree of mosaicism is low in the resulting animals, and that proviruses are located preferentially in genes likely to be active at the time of infection.

MATERIALS AND METHODS

Lentiviral vector-mediated transgenesis. We generated transgenic mice by perivitelline injection of fertilized oocytes, as described previously (13). Briefly, the hybrid strain B6D2G1 derived from C57BL/6JxDBA2J mice (Charles River, France) was used as an egg donor. Superovulation was induced by intraperitoneal injection of five B6D2G1 females with 10 IU of pregnant mare serum (Sigma, Buchs, Switzerland). Forty-six hours later, a second intraperitoneal injection of 10 IU of human chorionic gonadotropin (Sigma) was performed before mice were mated with B6D2G1 males. Sixteen hours later, oocytes were harvested, injected in the perivitelline space with a highly concentrated vector stock (5 × 10⁸ to 1 × 10⁹ HeLa-transducing units/ml), and kept in culture overnight at 37°C and 5% CO₂ in KSOM medium (MR-121; Specialty Media). Embryos that had reached the two-cell stage were then placed in the ampulla of foster NMRI mothers (eight embryos per ampulla). All vectors used in this study were previously described (27). Genotyping of the offspring was done by PCR using vector-specific primers (forward primer, 5'-TATGTTGCTCCTTTTACG CTATGTG-3'; reverse primer, 5'-CGACAACACCACGGAATTGT-3').

LAM-PCR. DNA of transgenic mice was purified by standard phenol-chloroform extraction and ethanol precipitation, and DNA of NIH 3T3 fibroblasts grown in Dulbecco's modified Eagle's medium–10% fetal calf serum (Invitrogen, Paisley, United Kingdom) was purified with a DNeasy extraction kit according to the manufacturer's recommendation (Qiagen, Hilden, Germany). Linear amplification-mediated (LAM)-PCR was carried out as described previously (18) with minor modifications. Five nanograms of genomic DNA was mixed in a 50-μl reaction volume with 1× Taq DNA polymerase buffer (Qiagen), a 200 μM concentration of the deoxynucleoside triphosphates (dNTPs) (Sigma, Buchs, Switzerland), a 2.5 nM concentration of oligonucleotides AD30 and AD31 (for all primers, see Table S3 in the supplemental material), and 2.5 U of Taq polymerase (Qiagen). Primers were extended after initial denaturation for 5 min at 94°C (hot start), followed by 50 cycles of 94°C for 1 min, 60°C for 45 s, and 72°C for 1.5 min, with a final extension at 72°C for 10 min. Dynal kilobaseBINDER beads (Invitrogen) were washed two times with 0.1% bovine serum albumin in phosphate-buffered saline, resuspended in 50 μl of binding buffer provided with the kit, and added to the PCR at a final concentration of 20 μl of beads per PCR. Extension products were captured for 1 h at room temperature under agitation and washed with water. Second strands were synthesized in 20-μl reaction mixtures containing 1× hexanucleotide buffer (Roche, Rotkreuz, Switzerland), 30 μM dNTPs, and 2 U of Klenow (Roche) for 1 h at 37°C. Beads were washed with water and digested in a 20-μl mixture containing 4 U of Tsp509I (New England Biolabs, Allschwil, Switzerland) for 1 h at 65°C. Beads were washed with water and ligated in a 10-μl reaction mixture containing 1× Fast-Link buffer (Epicenter, Dottikon, Switzerland), 1 mM ATP, 2 μl of AD25/AD26 linker cassette, and 2 U of Fast-Link ligase for 5 min at room temperature. Beads were washed with water and denatured for 10 min at room temperature with 5 μl of 0.1 M NaOH. Two microliters of this LAM product was exponentially amplified in 50-μl reaction mixtures containing 1× Taq DNA polymerase buffer (Qiagen), 200 μM dNTPs (Sigma), 500 nM concentrations of oligonucleotides AD27 and AD32, and 5 U of Taq polymerase (Qiagen). Primers were extended after initial denaturation for 3 min at 94°C (hot start) followed by 35 cycles of 94°C for 45 min,

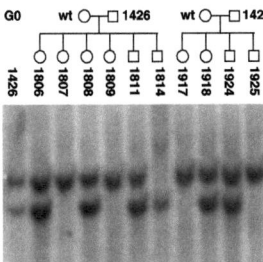

FIG. 2. Lentiviral vector transmission detected by Southern blotting. A Southern blot of tail DNA of G1 offspring. The founder animal (G0, animal 1426) carried two copies of the pWPTS provirus. Crossing the G0 animal with a wild-type (wt) animal gave a total of 20 pups with 10 (50%) transgenic animals. Circles and squares represent males and females, respectively.

60°C for 45 min, and 72°C for 45 s, with a final extension at 72°C for 10 min. One microliter of this PCR product was amplified in a 50-μl reaction mixture with 1× Taq DNA polymerase buffer (Qiagen), 200 μM dNTPs (Sigma), 500 nM AD33 (oligonucleotide), 400 nM AD28, 100 nM AD62, and 5 U of Taq polymerase (Qiagen). One microliter of the final PCR product was mixed with 0.5 μl of ROX GeneScan standard (Applied Biosystems, Switzerland) and 8.5 μl of distilled formamide (Applied Biosystems) and denatured for 2 min at 95°C. PCRs were separated on a 3100 sequencer (Applied Biosystems) and analyzed with the GeneScan software.

Cloning, sequencing, and annotation of LAM-PCR products. PCRs were purified with a Nucleobond II kit (Macherey-Nagel, Switzerland) and eluted in 30 μl of 5 mM Tris-HCl, pH 8.0. Fifteen microliters of this eluate was digested overnight with 5 U of NarI (NEB) in a 20-μl reaction volume at 37°C. Of this digest, 0.6 μl was mixed in 96-well plates with 0.5 μl of pCR4-TOPO (Invitrogen) and 0.4 μl of salt solution in a final volume of 2.3 μl. After incubation for 5 min at room temperature, reaction mixtures were heat shocked into DH5α cells provided with the kit (Invitrogen). Colonies were picked into 96-well plates and sequenced at GATC Biotech, Konstanz, Germany. Sequences were extracted from chromatograms using phred (3). Vector and HIV-contaminating sequences plus U5 and LC fragments were identified with BLAT (12) and removed prior to annotation. Mouse repeats in the cleaned sequences were identified and masked with RepeatMasker (A. F. A. Smit, R. Hubley, and P. Green, unpublished data). The location of each cleaned, masked sequence in the mouse genome (NCBIm34 assembly) was determined with the Megablast program (32) using a word length of 24. The annotation procedure was automated using a series of ad hoc Perl scripts. Gene-relative mappings were determined using the ENSEMBL database (http://oct2006.archive.ensembl.org/). We defined genes as transcription units annotated in the ENSEMBL database; data tables were assembled in Open-Office, version 2.0, and statistical analysis was performed with R or PRISM (version 4.0) software.

ISS-PCR. Integration site-specific PCRs (ISS-PCRs) were exponentially amplified in 25-μl reaction mixtures containing 100 ng of DNA, 1.5× Taq Polymerase buffer (Qiagen), 200 μM dNTPs (Promega), 0.8 μg of bovine serum albumin (NEB), 25 mmol MgCl$_2$ (Qiagen), 5 U of HotStart Taq polymerase (Qiagen), and 200 nM concentrations of each primer. The PCR started with an initial activation step of 95°C for 15 min (hot start), followed by 10 cycles of 94°C for 45 s, 60°C (with a change of −1°C per cycle) for 45 s, and 72°C for 1 min (touchdown); this program was followed by 30 cycles of 94°C for 45 s, 50°C for 45 s, and 72°C for 1 min, with a final extension at 72°C for 10 min. Five milliliters of loading buffer (6×) was added to each PCR, and 15 μl was run on a 0.8% agarose gel for about 30 min at 80V before analysis under UV light.

RNA expression measurements. NIH 3T3 fibroblasts were cultured in Dulbecco's modified Eagle's medium–10% fetal calf serum (Invitrogen) at 37°C in 5% CO$_2$. Oct4-GiP (kind gift A. Smith, Edinburgh, United Kingdom) embryonic stem (ES) cells were cultured as described previously (31) in the presence of 500 ng of puromycin (Sigma)/ml at 37°C in 10% CO$_2$. RNA was isolated with Trizol (Invitrogen) and ethanol precipitation according to standard procedures; cDNA was synthesized with hexanucleotides according to the manufacturer's recommendation using a SuperScript III first-strand cDNA synthesis system (Invitrogen). Fifty unfertilized eggs or two-cell embryos were resuspended in 1 μl of

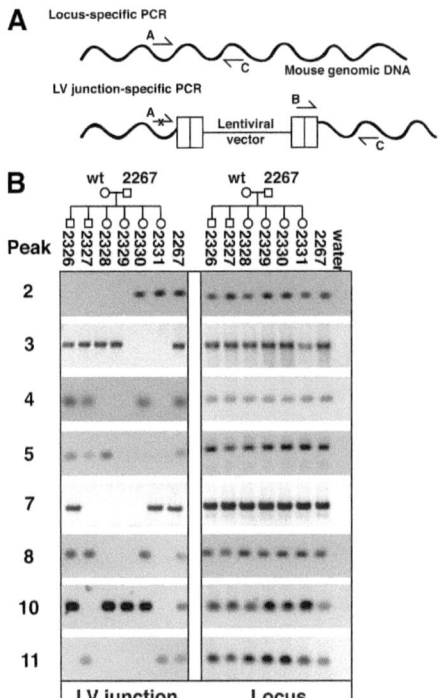

FIG. 3. Lentivirus transmission detected by ISS-PCR. (A) Scheme of primer sets used for ISS-PCR on tail DNA targeting the integrated provirus or the integration site in G1. Primer set A plus C surrounds the lentivirus integration site (locus), and primer set B plus C targets the lentiviral vector and the downstream genome sequence (junction). (B) PCR analysis of the offspring from mouse 2267 crossed with a wild-type (wt) animal. LV, lentivirus.

RNase Out and 10 μl of resuspension buffer (SuperScript III CellsDirect cDNA synthesis system; Invitrogen) and denatured for 10 min at 75°C. DNase digestion was carried out according to the manufacturer's instructions, and 2 μl of 50 ng/μl hexamer was added with 1 μl of dNTPs. Reaction mixtures were denatured at 70°C for 5 min, and the remaining reagents were added as indicated in the protocol. Reaction mixtures were left for 10 min at 25°C before reverse transcription. RNase H-digested cDNAs were used for quantitative PCR. The expression of each gene was assayed in triplicate in a total volume of 5 μl containing 1× Power Sybr (Applied Biosystems), a 200 nM concentration of each gene-specific primer pair (see Table S3 in the supplemental material), and diluted cDNA (cultured cells, 1:17; embryonic cDNA, 1:2.6). To verify specificity, each PCR was followed by a melting curve analysis, and samples lacking reverse transcriptase were run in parallel. The increase in fluorescence was analyzed with SDS software, version 2.2.2, (Applied Biosystems). For all amplification plots, the baseline data were set with the automatic cycle threshold function available with SDS, version 2.2.2, calculating the optimal baseline range and threshold values by using the AutoCt algorithm (SDS version 2.2 user's manual, Applied Biosystems, Foster City, CA). A mean quantity was calculated from triplicate PCRs for each sample, and this quantity was normalized to two similarly measured quantities of normalization genes as described previously (24). Normalized quantities were averaged for three replicates for each data point and are represented as the means ± standard deviations (SD). The highest normalized relative

TABLE 1. Integration sites of G0 mouse 2267 outside annotated genes

Integrant identifier	Chromosome	Position (nt)	Strand	Distance to nearest gene (nt)	Sense of transcription	ENSEMBL identifier
2267-132D	1	23905241	+	101,830	Upstream	ENSMUSG00000026156
2267-132R3	X	46760215	+	33,008	Upstream	ENSMUSG00000055653
2267-132F	10	103196281	+	45,568	Downstream	ENSMUSG00000019892
2267-132R2	2	150665634	+	165,266	Upstream	ENSMUSG00000048918
2267-132C	15	69704246	−	578,594	Downstream	ENSMUSG00000022332
2267-132D	1	23905241	+	101,830	Upstream	ENSMUSG00000026156

quantity was arbitrarily given a value of 1.0. Relative changes were calculated from the quotient of the means of these normalized quantities and are reported as means ± SD.

RESULTS

Timing lentiviral vector integration in germ cell precursors. The degree of mosaicism of mice obtained by lentivector-mediated transgenesis reflects the timing of integration in primary blastomeres. As a first assessment of this parameter, we injected an enhanced green fluorescent protein (eGFP)-expressing vector (Fig. 1A, pWPTS) into the perivitelline space of fertilized mouse oocytes and let the resulting embryos develop in vitro to the blastocyst stage. Upon fluorescence microscopy examination, both the inner cell mass and the trophectoderm revealed uniformly high levels of eGFP expression (Fig. 1B). While this result indicated that transcription proceeded efficiently from the EF1α (elongation factor 1α) promoter contained in this vector, it did not differentiate the rapid integration of one or more proviruses into the zygote from the delayed integration of multiple proviruses in later cells or a combination thereof. Measuring integration kinetics directly was difficult due to the small number of cells concerned. We therefore used an indirect yet highly quantitative approach to define this parameter. For this, we proceeded to a large-scale determination of the rates of G0 to G1 transmission of individual integrants, using a combination of Southern blotting and ISS-PCR. An example of Southern blotting-based analysis is depicted in Fig. 2. Tail DNA from the G0 mouse 1426 generated with the pLV-tTRKRAB-red vector (Fig. 1A) revealed that this animal harbored two proviruses. Crossing this mouse with a wild-type animal produced a G1 progeny of 20 members, out of which half were transgenic, as determined by PCR amplification of tail DNA with vector-specific primers (data not shown). Southern blot analysis of this transgenic offspring revealed that the two proviruses had overall rates of germ line transmission of 45% and 30%, respectively.

Southern blotting becomes more difficult to interpret when a mouse harbors a large number of proviruses. Thus, to assess lentivirus transmission more unequivocally, we used ISS-PCR to trace lentiviral integrants in G1 mice. Analysis of the 2267 family is representative of the results obtained by this technique (Fig. 3). We first mapped lentivirus integration sites in G0 animals by LAM-PCR (18). Integration sites 4, 5, and 8 were located outside of annotated genes (Table 1). Proviruses 2 and 11 were oriented in antisense or sense, respectively, with respect to the transcriptional orientation of the target gene (Table 2). Three integrants were of a repetitive nature (Table 3). We then designed for each integration site a set of three primers, allowing a distinction between genomic loci that either did or did not contain the integrant (Fig. 3A). For each locus, we performed two PCR amplifications in parallel, one specific for the host sequences flanking the integration site (locus PCR) and the other across the junction between the 3′ end of the provirus and the host DNA (junction PCR) (Fig. 3B). The combined results of these two PCRs indicated unequivocally whether a provirus was present in a mouse.

These techniques in hand, we generated 11 transgenic founders through as many independent sessions of injection; five carried the pLV-tTRKRAB-red vector, and six carried the pRRL-GFP vector (Fig. 1A). These animals were crossed with a wild-type animal, yielding a total of 111 pups. Seventy proviral insertions were mapped in the G0 mice, and 255 were mapped in the G1 mice. Overall, the average rate of transmission of individual proviruses was 44% (Fig. 4A). When mice were grouped according to the vector used, germ line transmission rates were 48% for pRRL-GFP and 34% for pLV-tTRKRAB-red (Fig. 4B). Of note, none of the vectors induced a drop in the size of the progeny in these or in other experiments, indicating that, as heterozygous provirus, none of the vectors exerted major phenotoxic effects that could have invalidated our genotypic analyses.

We also characterized the distribution of lentiviral integrants in G2 animals obtained by G1-G0 backcrossing of the 2267 lineage by ISS-PCR. Eight integrants could be success-

TABLE 2. Integration sites of G0 mouse 2267 inside annotated genes

Integrant identifier	Chromosome	Position (nt)	Strand	Sense of TU[a]	ENSEMBL identifier	Gene[b]
2267-132A	5	61423827	+	−	ENSMUSG00000037999	Centd1
2267-132E	1	8362904	+	−	ENSMUSG00000067894	No description
2267-132I	3	58744450	−	+	ENSMUSG00000056476	Med12l
2267-132G	4	8753066	−	+	ENSMUSG00000050506	No description
2267-132H	4	10990240	−	−	ENSMUSG00000050323	XP_131300

[a] TU, transcription unit.
[b] From the Mouse Genome Informatics database.

TABLE 3. Integration sites of G0 mouse 2267 in repeats

Integrant identifier	Class	Repeat
2267-132R1	LTR/ERVL[a]	MERVL[b]
2267-132R2	LTR/ERVK[a]	IAPEz-int
2267-132R3	LINE/L1	Lx7

[a] ERVL/K, endogenous retrovirus repeat family.
[b] MERVL, mouse endogenous retrovirus repeat family.

fully amplified using this technique. In the G2 animals, integrants 2, 4, 5, 8, and 11 yielded a positive result by junction PCR and a negative result by locus PCR, indicating that the corresponding provirus was present in both alleles (Fig. 5A). Noteworthy, the frequency of homozygous integrants in G2 animals positively correlated with the number of proviral copies in G1 animals ($r^2 = 0.99$), reaching an overall value of 7.69% (8/104) in this particular case, which is significantly lower than expected from the 25% of a purely Mendelian

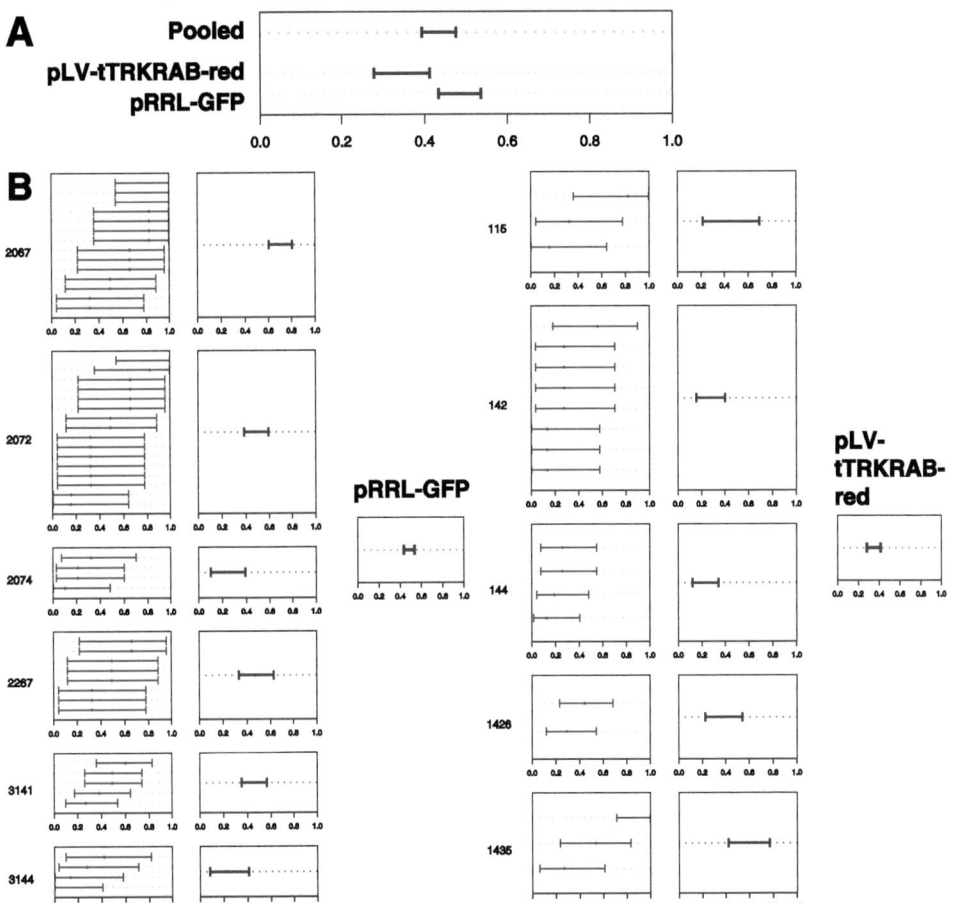

FIG. 4. Frequency of G0-to-G1 transmission of lentiviral proviruses. (A) All integrants were pooled to obtain a global rate of transmission of lentiviral vector. Data are given for pooled integrants containing either pLV-tTRKRAB-red or pRRL-GFP from transgenic mice. (B) Point estimates represent the actual proportion of transmission for each integrant. Error bars indicate the 95% confidence interval obtained. The observations corresponding to different integrants in the same founder were pooled, assuming an equal probability of transmission for all integrants within the founder; the pooled estimates and their associated confidence intervals are shown for each family. The confidence intervals are narrower than those obtained for single integrants since they are based on larger sets of data. Finally, all the integrants of founders carrying the same promoter were pooled to obtain an average rate of transmission of individual integrants from this vector, with confidence interval.

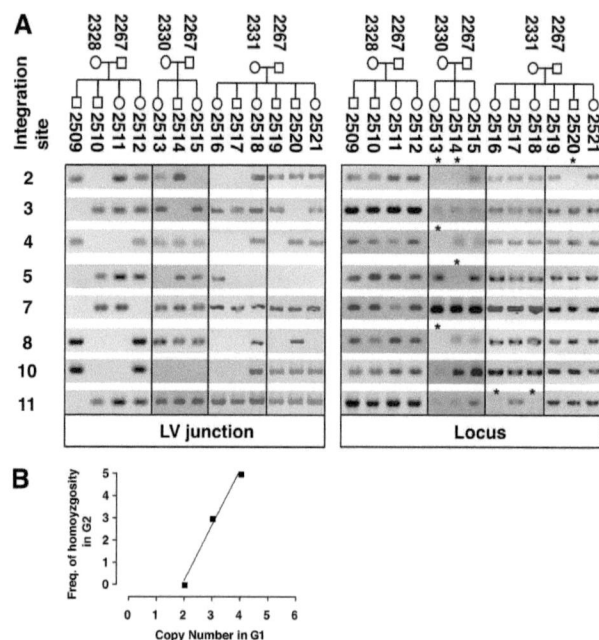

FIG. 5. Transmission of lentiviral vectors to G2 mice. (A) G2 animals obtained from crossing G0 animal 2267 with three G1 animals. G2 animals were analyzed by the same PCR as described in the legend of Fig. 3. The asterisks mark gene-specific PCRs that failed to amplify the wild-type locus (mice carrying lentiviral vectors in both alleles). Every PCR was run with DNA from the founder animal amplifying all integration sites and a negative control from a nontransgenic animal (not shown). (B) The frequency (Freq.) of homozygous transmission of lentivirus integration sites 2, 4, 5, 8, and 11 in G2 animals correlates with the copy number of lentiviral vectors detected in the G1 animals. LV, lentivirus.

transmission. However, there was no difference in the G1 transmission frequency of proviruses that did or did not reach homozygosity in G2 animals (Fig. 3), suggesting that these proviruses were not toxic in the heterozygous state.

Integration site selection. We then examined the in vivo integration site selection in lentivirus transgenic mice at a genomic level. We limited our mapping effort to LAM-PCR-generated amplicons containing at least 20 nucleotides (nt) of genomic sequence in addition to the 120 nt derived from the viral long terminal repeat (LTR) and linker cassettes, mapping successfully 239 sites in 49 G0 animals. We compared this integration data set to that of 108 lentiviral integrants obtained by transduction of murine 3T3 fibroblasts (see Tables S1 and S2 in the supplemental material). Proviruses were detectable in all chromosomes except Y (Fig. 6A). The likelihood of integration inside a gene was 1.75- and 1.88-fold higher in transgenic mice and 3T3 fibroblasts, respectively, than expected from the distribution of annotated genes in the mouse genome ($P_{mice} = 3.03e^{-09}$; $P_{3T3} = 5.55e^{-16}$) (Fig. 6B). Integration was not influenced by the transcriptional orientation of the target gene (Fig. 6C) (sense orientation, 51.7%; antisense orientation, 48.3%), but proviruses seemed to cluster around 20 kb downstream of the transcriptional start site of annotated genes (Fig. 6D). To analyze this pattern in more detail, we divided the distance of the lentiviral integration site to the transcriptional start site by the size of the target gene. This revealed a relative enrichment of integrants in the middle of the genes (mean value ± SD of 0.527 ± 0.255 for transgenic mice and 0.523 ± 0.274 for 3T3 fibroblasts). To compare these results to data previously obtained in human cells, we similarly analyzed 124 randomly picked, previously mapped HIV-1 integration sites in human SupT1 cells (19). In this collection as well, we observed the accumulation of lentiviral integrants in the middle of the genes (distance from transcription start/length of transcribed region, 0.500 ± 0.281).

One characteristic feature of mammalian genomes is the high content of repetitive elements. The mouse genome harbors three major classes of repeats: long interspersed nuclear elements (LINEs), short interspersed nuclear elements, and LTRs (11). We found that the percentage of integration into repeats closely corresponded to their relative abundance in the mouse genome (36.0% versus 38.0%) (26). Integration into repeats was slightly lower in 3T3 fibroblasts (30.8%), but the difference between these cells and cells of transgenic animals was not statistically significant. Comparison of the fraction of lentiviral vectors integrated into different repeat classes

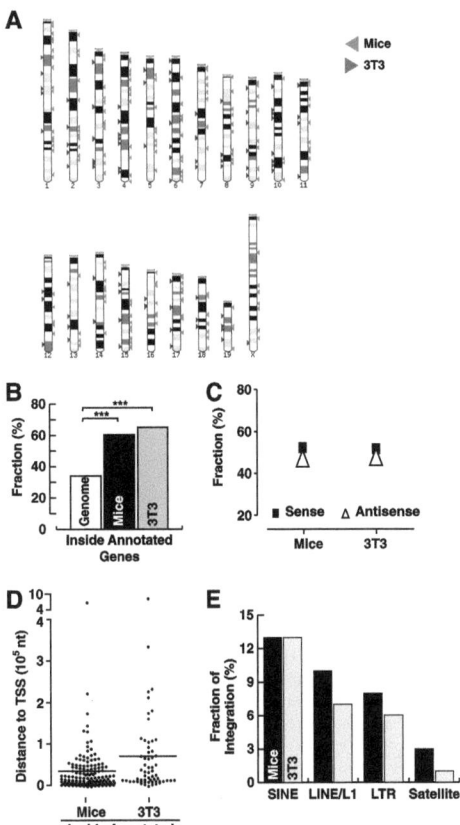

FIG. 6. Distribution of lentiviral integration sites in the mouse genome. (A) Chromosomal distribution of in vivo lentiviral integration sites in transgenic mice. (B) The fraction of lentiviral vectors inside a gene was determined in transgenic mice and 3T3 fibroblasts with ENSEMBL, version 42, as a reference. To calculate P values, we applied a binomial distribution where the expected probability was taken from the whole-genome fractions. The P values were 4.85^{-12} for integration sites in transgenic mice (∗∗∗) and 3.75^{-8} for 3T3 fibroblasts (∗∗). (C) Orientation of lentiviral vectors inside a gene was compared to the transcriptional orientation of the target gene in transgenic mice and 3T3 fibroblasts. (D) The absolute distance of the lentiviral vector to the transcriptional start site (TSS) was determined in transgenic mice and 3T3 fibroblasts. (E) The fraction of integration sites in LINE/L1, endogenous retroviruses (LTRs), and short interspersed nuclear elements (SINE) in 3T3 fibroblasts and transgenic mice was divided by the fraction of these repeats in the mouse genome.

showed a slight preference for LTR, LINE/L1, and satellite repeats in the transgenic mice, possibly contributing to this marginal difference (Fig. 6E).

Integration appears to favor genes expressed during early embryogenesis. In order to test whether integration favored genes transcriptionally active during the preimplantation stages of the embryo, as previously observed in adult cells, we used quantitative PCR to compare the expression patterns of 10 randomly selected lentivirus target genes in two-cell embryos, ES cells, and 3T3 fibroblasts (Fig. 7A). Expression of these genes in two-cell embryos was from 2 to 42 times higher than that of housekeeping genes taken as controls (left panel). In ES cells and 3T3 fibroblasts, their expression was generally lower than in two-cell embryos (Fig. 7A), but this in part reflected higher average levels of RNA transcripts in the latter cells (9.5-fold difference; one-way analysis of variance, $P <$ 0.0001) (Fig. 7B). Additionally, we tested the impact of maternal RNA expression levels by comparing the expression of eight lentivirus target genes in unfertilized oocytes with expression in two-cell embryos. Two of the genes (5830435K17Rik and Bbs4) had similar expression levels in both settings, suggesting that their transcripts might be predominantly of maternal origin (Fig. 7C). In contrast, expression levels of the remaining six target genes were higher in two-cell embryos than in unfertilized oocytes.

DISCUSSION

PCR-based analyses of the kinetics of lentivirus/HIV integration previously revealed that, in human T-lymphoid cell lines, integration starts 4 h after infection and reaches its maximum after 16 h (22). Due to the low abundance of material at hand following infection of zygotes, we could not define this parameter directly in this setting. Instead, we examined the rates of transmission of individual proviruses from G0 transgenic mice to their G1 progeny. The overall rate of transmission of 44% for individual proviruses suggests that they were most often established at the one-cell stage after the S phase or at the two-cell stage before the S phase, since integration prior to S phase would transmit the provirus to both daughter cells, while integration after the S phase would transmit it to only one daughter cell. Considering the approximately 12-h division time of early blastomeres typical of our experimental conditions, the kinetics of lentivirus integration are thus not greatly delayed in these cells compared to T-lymphoid cells. A consequence is that the degree of mosaicism for individual integrants is minimal in transgenic mice obtained through this technique. This contrasts with data obtained in transgenic rats similarly generated, where a far higher degree of mosaicism was observed (23). While species-specific differences are possible, only a side-by-side comparison of similar vector preparations used to infect mouse and rat oocytes in parallel would properly address this question.

We also determined the genomic distribution of the proviral integrants generated by lentivector-mediated transgenesis. Following LAM-PCR-mediated amplification and sequencing of the host genome-provirus junctions, we could successfully locate more than 85% of the integration sites using a Perl script, which automatically removes cloning vector sequences, masks repetitive elements, and aligns the remaining polynucleotidic stretches with the mouse genome. This stepwise procedure enabled us to assign LAM-PCR-generated sequences to the mouse genome even when part of the amplicon was constituted by repetitive sequences, a point verified by ISS-PCR. This latter method, which dually targets the provi-

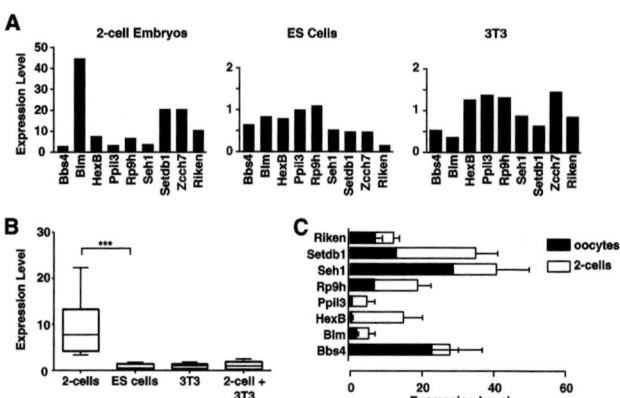

FIG. 7. Expression of lentivirus target genes in different mouse tissues. Transcript levels of lentivirus target genes were determined by quantitative PCR cDNAs synthesized on two-cell embryos, ES cells, and 3T3 fibroblasts RNA. PCR on cDNA synthesized without reverse transcriptase were negative (not shown). Expression levels were calculated relative to the function of three normalization genes included in each PCR. All PCRs were performed in triplicate. (A) Expression levels of 10 arbitrarily chosen lentivirus target genes in the indicated tissues. Shown are mean values of three independent experiments. (B) Box plot of the expression levels determined in panel A plus a control in which RNA isolated from two-cell embryos mixed with 10 ng of 3T3 fibroblast RNA served as templates for the cDNA synthesis. Expression levels determined in two-cell embryos and ES cells were compared by one-way analysis of variance (***, $P < 0.0001$). (C) Expression levels of eight lentivirus target genes in unfertilized oocytes and two-cell embryos. Shown are mean values ± standard errors of two independent experiments.

rus-genome junction and the targeted locus, was previously used to trace retrovirally marked repopulating hematopoietic stem cells. Here, it allowed us to identify unequivocally transgenic G2 mice that were homozygous for specific lentiviral integrants following G0-G1 crosses. The observed frequency of homozygosity was below the 25% expected from a purely Mendelian mode of transmission. Considering the rapid kinetics of integration, it is unlikely that these non-Mendelian transmission rates reflect mosaicism in the germ line. Rather, some of the homozygous G2 mice must be nonviable due to the target gene inactivation potential of retrovirus integrants. However, the normal rates of G1 representation of proviruses that did not achieve homozygosity in G2 suggest an absence of toxicity in the heterozygous state. It remains that our series is very small and that a much larger study would certainly be needed to probe this issue and to confirm that homozygous lentiviral integrants are significantly counter-selected due to gene inactivation.

It was previously noted that the lentiviruses HIV, simian immunodeficiency virus, equine infectious anemia virus, and feline immunodeficiency virus and the vectors derived thereof exhibit similar integration patterns in human, monkey, and murine cells (1, 2, 6, 7, 10). Here, we extend the analysis to transgenic mice generated by infection of fertilized oocytes. We found that, in this case, HIV-derived lentiviral integrants favor genes, where they integrate with a tendency for the middle of the transcribed region, a trend already noted in human cells. One explanation could be that genes form a loop, with the transcriptional start and termination sites serving as bridging points and the tip of the loop protruding to the outside, which makes it more accessible for integration. Alternatively, occupancy of the transcriptional start and termination regions by regulatory proteins might interfere with this process. However, the accumulation of MLV integrants within or near promoters makes either one of these simple models unlikely. Instead, it is tempting to postulate that retroviral preintegration complexes interact with the RNA polymerase II holoenzyme and associated proteins and/or recognize specific histone modifications. Histone 3 dimethylation at lysine 4 correlates with active transcription and accumulates in the middle of genes, as do lentiviral integrants (17). In contrast, histone 3 monomethylation at lysine 4 and diacetylation at lysine 14 cluster at the transcriptional start sites, reminiscent of the MLV integration pattern. Thus, chromatin modifications or factors catalyzing these modifications might act as key players in the viral DNA-host genome interface, as recently suggested (25).

We observed a subtle difference in the integration patterns of lentiviral vectors in 3T3 fibroblasts and transgenic mice, with a slightly higher frequency of integration into repeats in the latter setting. Although this difference was statistically not significant, it might reflect the elevated transcriptional activity of repetitive elements in preimplantation embryos (15, 16, 21). In support of this model, we found that genes targeted by the lentiviral integrants in transgenic mice generally had higher levels of expression in two-cell embryos than in adult tissues. However, the constantly evolving picture of expressed regions of the genome, now known to encompass far more than conventional genes, as well as evidence indicating that genes that are poised for activation may share chromatin marks with actively transcribed genes, call for caution in establishing overly strict correlations, based on monomethylation at lysine 4, between "gene expression" and retroviral integration site selection.

ACKNOWLEDGMENTS

We thank S. Verp, M. Arcangeli, S. Liao, and J. Jakobsson (EPFL) for technical assistance or the gift of reagents; M. Docquier, C. Delucinge, and P. Descombes (NCCR Frontiers in Genetics) for help with the genomics analyses; C. Prinz and M. Schmidt (University of Freiburg, Germany) for teaching us LAM-PCR; and M. Delorenzi (Swiss Institute of Bioinformatics) for advice on the statistics.

This work was supported by the European Union as part of the 6th Framework Program CONSERT project and by the Swiss National Science Foundation.

The authors declare that they have no conflict of interests.

REFERENCES

1. **Beard, B. C., D. Dickerson, K. Beebe, C. Gooch, J. Fletcher, T. Okbinoglu, D. G. Miller, M. A. Jacobs, R. Kaul, H. P. Kiem, and G. D. Trobridge.** 2007. Comparison of HIV-derived lentiviral and MLV-based gammaretroviral vector integration sites in primate repopulating cells. Mol. Ther. **15:**1356–1365.
2. **Bushman, F., M. Lewinski, A. Ciuffi, S. Barr, J. Leipzig, S. Hannenhalli, and C. Hoffmann.** 2005. Genome-wide analysis of retroviral DNA integration. Nature Rev. Microbiol. **3:**848–858.
3. **Ewing, B., L. Hillier, M. C. Wendl, and P. Green.** 1998. Base-calling of automated sequencer traces using PHRED. I. Accuracy assessment. Genome Res. **8:**175–185.
4. **Fassler, R.** 2004. Lentiviral transgene vectors. EMBO Rep. **5:**28–29.
5. **Gordon, J. W., G. A. Scangos, D. J. Plotkin, J. A. Barbosa, and F. H. Ruddle.** 1980. Genetic transformation of mouse embryos by microinjection of purified DNA. Proc. Natl. Acad. Sci. USA **77:**7380–7384.
6. **Hacker, C. V., C. A. Vink, T. W. Wardell, S. Lee, P. Treasure, S. M. Kingsman, K. A. Mitrophanous, and J. E. Miskin.** 2006. The integration profile of EIAV-based vectors. Mol. Ther. **14:**536–545.
7. **Hematti, P., B.-K. Hong, C. Ferguson, R. Adler, H. Hanawa, S. Sellers, I. E. Holt, C. E. Eckfeldt, Y. Sharma, M. Schmidt, C. von Kalle, D. A. Persons, E. M. Billings, C. M. Verfaillie, A. W. Nienhuis, T. G. Wolfsberg, C. E. Dunbar, and B. Calmels.** 2004. Distinct genomic integration of MLV and SIV vectors in primate hematopoietic stem and progenitor cells. PLoS Biol. **2:**e423.
8. **Hofmann, A., B. Kessler, S. Ewerling, A. Kabermann, G. Brem, E. Wolf, and A. Pfeifer.** 2006. Epigenetic regulation of lentiviral transgene vectors in a large animal model. Mol. Ther. **13:**59–66.
9. **Jahner, D., H. Stuhlmann, C. L. Stewart, K. Harbers, J. Lohler, I. Simon, and R. Jaenisch.** 1982. De novo methylation and expression of retroviral genomes during mouse embryogenesis. Nature **298:**623–628.
10. **Kang, Y., C. J. Moressi, T. E. Scheetz, L. Xie, D. T. Tran, L. Casavant, P. Ak, C. J. Benham, B. L. Davidson, and P. B. McCray, Jr.** 2006. Integration site choice of a feline immunodeficiency virus vector. J. Virol. **80:**8820–8823.
11. **Kazazian, H. H., Jr.** 2004. Mobile elements: drivers of genome evolution. Science **303:**1626–1632.
12. **Kent, W. J.** 2002. BLAT–the BLAST-like alignment tool. Genome Res. **12:**656–664.
13. **Lois, C., E. J. Hong, S. Pease, E. J. Brown, and D. Baltimore.** 2002. Germline transmission and tissue-specific expression of transgenes delivered by lentiviral vectors. Science **295:**868–872.
14. **Mitchell, R. S., B. F. Beitzel, A. R. Schroder, P. Shinn, H. Chen, C. C. Berry, J. R. Ecker, and F. D. Bushman.** 2004. Retroviral DNA integration: ASLV, HIV, and MLV show distinct target site preferences. PLoS Biol. **2:**E234.
15. **Ostertag, E. M., R. J. DeBerardinis, J. L. Goodier, Y. Zhang, N. Yang, G. L. Gerton, and H. H. Kazazian, Jr.** 2002. A mouse model of human L1 retrotransposition. Nat. Genet. **32:**655–660.
16. **Peaston, A. E., A. V. Evsikov, J. H. Graber, W. N. de Vries, A. E. Holbrook, D. Solter, and B. B. Knowles.** 2004. Retrotransposons regulate host genes in mouse oocytes and preimplantation embryos. Dev. Cell **7:**597–606.
17. **Pokholok, D. K., C. T. Harbison, S. Levine, M. Cole, N. M. Hannett, T. I. Lee, G. W. Bell, K. Walker, P. A. Rolfe, E. Herbolsheimer, J. Zeitlinger, F. Lewitter, D. K. Gifford, and R. A. Young.** 2005. Genome-wide map of nucleosome acetylation and methylation in yeast. Cell **122:**517–527.
18. **Schmidt, M., P. Zickler, G. Hoffmann, S. Haas, M. Wissler, A. Muessig, J. F. Tisdale, K. Kuramoto, R. G. Andrews, T. Wu, H. P. Kiem, C. E. Dunbar, and C. von Kalle.** 2002. Polyclonal long-term repopulating stem cell clones in a primate model. Blood **100:**2737–2743.
19. **Schroder, A. R., P. Shinn, H. Chen, C. Berry, J. R. Ecker, and F. Bushman.** 2002. HIV-1 integration in the human genome favors active genes and local hotspots. Cell **110:**521–529.
20. **Tiscornia, G., O. Singer, M. Ikawa, and I. M. Verma.** 2003. A general method for gene knockdown in mice by using lentiviral vectors expressing small interfering RNA. Proc. Natl. Acad. Sci. USA **100:**1844–1848.
21. **Trelogan, S. A., and S. L. Martin.** 1995. Tightly regulated, developmentally specific expression of the first open reading frame from LINE-1 during mouse embryogenesis. Proc. Natl. Acad. Sci. USA **92:**1520–1524.
22. **Vandegraaff, N., R. Kumar, C. J. Burrell, and P. Li.** 2001. Kinetics of human immunodeficiency virus type 1 (HIV) DNA integration in acutely infected cells as determined using a novel assay for detection of integrated HIV DNA. J. Virol. **75:**11253–11260.
23. **van den Brandt, J., D. Wang, S.-H. Kwon, M. Heinkelein, and H. M. Reichardt.** 2004. Lentivirally generated eGFP-transgenic rats allow efficient cell tracking in vivo. Genesis **39:**94–99.
24. **Vandesompele, J., K. De Preter, F. Pattyn, B. Poppe, N. Van Roy, A. De Paepe, and F. Speleman.** 2002. Accurate normalization of real-time quantitative RT-PCR data by geometric averaging of multiple internal control genes. Genome Biol **3:**research0034.1–0034.11. http://genomebiology.com/2002/3/7/research/0034.
25. **Wang, G. P., A. Ciuffi, J. Leipzig, C. C. Berry, and F. D. Bushman.** 2007. HIV integration site selection: analysis by massively parallel pyrosequencing reveals association with epigenetic modifications. Genome Res. **17:**1186–1194.
26. **Waterston, R. H., K. Lindblad-Toh, E. Birney, J. Rogers, J. F. Abril, P. Agarwal, R. Agarwala, R. Ainscough, M. Alexandersson, P. An, S. E. Antonarakis, J. Attwood, R. Baertsch, J. Bailey, K. Barlow, S. Beck, E. Berry, B. Birren, T. Bloom, P. Bork, M. Botcherby, N. Bray, M. R. Brent, D. G. Brown, S. D. Brown, C. Bult, J. Burton, J. Butler, R. D. Campbell, P. Carninci, S. Cawley, F. Chiaromonte, A. T. Chinwalla, D. M. Church, M. Clamp, C. Clee, F. S. Collins, L. L. Cook, R. R. Copley, A. Coulson, O. Couronne, J. Cuff, V. Curwen, T. Cutts, M. Daly, R. David, J. Davies, K. D. Delehaunty, J. Deri, E. T. Dermitzakis, C. Dewey, N. J. Dickens, M. Diekhans, S. Dodge, I. Dubchak, D. M. Dunn, S. R. Eddy, L. Elnitski, R. D. Emes, P. Eswara, E. Eyras, A. Felsenfeld, G. A. Fewell, P. Flicek, K. Foley, W. N. Frankel, L. A. Fulton, R. S. Fulton, T. S. Furey, D. Gage, R. A. Gibbs, G. Glusman, S. Gnerre, N. Goldman, L. Goodstadt, D. Grafham, T. A. Graves, E. D. Green, S. Gregory, R. Guigo, M. Guyer, R. C. Hardison, D. Haussler, Y. Hayashizaki, L. W. Hillier, A. Hinrichs, W. Hlavina, T. Holzer, F. Hsu, A. Hua, T. Hubbard, A. Hunt, I. Jackson, D. B. Jaffe, L. S. Johnson, M. Jones, T. A. Jones, A. Joy, M. Kamal, E. K. Karlsson, et al.** 2002. Initial sequencing and comparative analysis of the mouse genome. Nature **420:**520–562.
27. **Wiznerowicz, M., and D. Trono.** 2003. Conditional suppression of cellular genes: lentivirus vector-mediated drug-inducible RNA interference. J. Virol. **77:**8957–8961.
28. **Wolf, D., F. Cammas, R. Losson, and S. P. Goff.** 2008. Primer binding site-dependent restriction of murine leukemia virus requires HP1 binding by TRIM28. J. Virol. **82:**4675–4679.
29. **Wolf, D., and S. P. Goff.** 2007. TRIM28 mediates primer binding site-targeted silencing of murine leukemia virus in embryonic cells. Cell **131:**46–57.
30. **Wu, X., Y. Li, B. Crise, and S. M. Burgess.** 2003. Transcription start regions in the human genome are favored targets for MLV integration. Science **300:**1749–1751.
31. **Ying, Q. L., J. Nichols, E. P. Evans, and A. G. Smith.** 2002. Changing potency by spontaneous fusion. Nature **416:**545–548.
32. **Zhang, Z., S. Schwartz, L. Wagner, and W. Miller.** 2000. A greedy algorithm for aligning DNA sequences. J. Comput. Biol. **7:**203–214.

Chapter 2. Genotypic features of lentiviral-derived transgenic mice

2.4 Conclusion

Numerous techniques can be used to insert exogenous DNA into the genome of living animals[2]. Broadly, we can separate two classes of experimental procedures: at one end stand the direct manipulations of the pronuclear genome and, at the other end, the gradual substitution of the genetic material of the embryo for that of ES cells[143]. The former generates animals carrying their original genome plus one exogenous sequence whereas the latter generates animals containing two genetically distinct cellular populations that will be completely skipped for that of the ES cells through one round of gametogenesis. Lentiviral vector-mediated transgenesis lies somewhere in the middle of the spectrum[152]. The unique potential of lentiviruses to integrate their DNA cargo into the cell genome combined with their broad host range can be used to target both zygotes and ES cells[159]. Retroviruses are not newcomers in the transgenic field. More than thirty years ago, MLV vectors were already used to generate transgenic animals[92]. However, some viral cis-acting sequences were methylated, preventing transgene expression[160]. It is not known whether this partly reflects differences in integration site selection, or solely results from the sequence-specific recruitment of epigenetic repressors, such as recently demonstrated for the primer-binding site (PBS)-dependent KAP1/TRIM28-mediated silencing of MLV vectors in embryonic stem cells[161]. As lentiviral vectors are less susceptible to methylation than MLV during embryogenesis, they were successfully used to generate animals expressing transgenes at high levels[101]. Interestingly, lentiviruses and gamma-retroviruses might have different intrinsic susceptibilities to silencing, perhaps as a consequence of their contrasting lifestyles. Whereas gamma-retroviruses rely on germline transmission as one form of spreading, lentiviruses rely exclusively on horizontal and non–germline vertical transfer. Thus, organisms might have evolved mechanisms to suppress the activity of endogenous gamma-retroviruses that would otherwise lead to their parasitic expansion in the genome. In contrast, such mechanisms might not target lentiviral sequences because endogenous lentiviruses have not been found in any mammalian genome. Alternatively, the lentiviral resistance to de novo methylation can lie in the large deletions of the U3 region of the viral 3' LTR, a known hotspot for methylation, during the development of lentiviral vector[38].

Chapter 2. Genotypic features of lentiviral-derived transgenic mice

The molecular mechanisms underlying the different sensitivity to methylation during embryogenesis are still not known. Nevertheless, lentiviral vector-mediated transgenesis opens new perspectives to manipulate the mammalian genome, including that of technically challenging species, such as pigs, sheep or cows and became an alternative to pronuclear injection of naked DNA. In the present work, we analyzed the genotypic features of lentiviral-mediated transgenic mice.

2.4.1 Lentiviral integration: a retrospective analysis

Transgenic animals are a valuable tool to analyze the physiological implication of the function or loss of function of a candidate gene. Due to the complexity of the in vivo setting, any technical problem that could interfere with the observed phenotype should be minimized. One major concern regarding lentiviral-mediated transgenesis is its potential to generate mosaic animals. Namely, the time of integration of lentiviral vector into host genome will directly determine the degree of mosaicism of the founder animal. The more delayed the integration, the more mosaic the resulting animal[162].

In this work, we designed experiments to assess the kinetic of lentiviral integration within the embryonic genome. In our preliminary analyses, we detected uniformly high levels of eGFP expression within the blastomeres at the blastocyst stage, following the injection of a lentiviral vector at the 1-cell stage. Although this result indicates that lentiviral vectors probably integrate the embryonic genome at an early stage and that the EF1alpha promoter contained in the vector used in these experiments is active at that stage, the analysis did not allow us to time lentiviral integration. Due to the low abundance of the material at hands, the use of conventional molecular analysis to quantify directly the timing of integration was not relevant. Therefore, we decided to analyze the kinetic of integration in an indirect yet highly quantitative way. For this, we proceeded to a large-scale determination of the rates of G0-to-G1 transmission of individual integrants. As the specification of primordial germ cells (PGC) in mammals is a relatively late event occurring after mid-gastrula, mammalian blastomeres contained within the ICM of blastocysts are still able to contribute to both the somatic and germ cells (Fig.8)[163,164]. Namely, in mice, PGCs first appear inside the extra-embryonic mesoderm at the posterior end of the primitive streak as a cluster of around 20 cells at d7.25[165]. Then, they undergo a rapid proliferation phase and migrate along the genital ridge reaching the gonads at d12.5. At d13.5 their number reaches up to about 26'000 (Fig.8). This is in contrast with other organisms such as Drosophila melanogaster, Caenorhabditis elegans or in Zebra fish[166, 167]. In these organisms, germ plasm (polar plasm) containing germ cell determinants is maternally accumulated and precisely localized in eggs. The blastomeres that inherit germ plasm will differentiate into germ cells. Therefore, the cell fate of early blastomeres is already set at day 0 and the decision relies exclusively on maternal cues. Therefore, we reasoned that

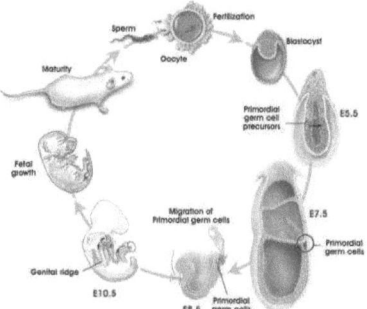

Fig. 8. Development of the primordial gem cells in mammals. (Derived from:"what are stem cells?".The official National Institutes of Health resource for stem cell research: stemcells.nih.gov/info/scireport/appendixA.asp.)

as early blastomeres contribute equally to the formation of primordial germ cells, the embryonic stage at which lentiviral vector integrates should have a direct impact on the rate of transmission. Thus, proviral segregation can be approximated as following mendelian laws: integration at the one-cell stage will lead to a 50% transmission in the progeny. Integration at the two-cell stage will decrease the rate of transmission to 25% and so on. We analyzed the individual transmission of 255 proviruses within the progeny of 11 founders crossed with wild type animals. We followed the different proviruses by Southern blot or integration site specific PCR (ISS PCR), a LAM based method that will be further discussed below. The statistical analysis gave a global rate of transmission of individual integrant from F0 to F1 of 0.435 (interval: 0.394 to 0.476). Thus, according to the classical laws of transmission, the integration is on average completed by the 2-cell stage. As the first division of the zygote occurs about 24 hours after fertilization, which takes place on a normal day-night cycle in an animal house (7am-5pm) at around 12pm and as the lentiviral injection is usually performed around 2pm, the time remaining for integration can be estimated to be 10-15 hours. This is in accordance with a recent study showing that lentiviral vector integration into cellular DNA can be detected as early as 4 hours post-infection, reaching its maximum at 16 hours[162]. The detailed analysis of the different colonies generated in our study showed different rates of transmission according to the lentiviral vector used. The pLV-tTRKRAB-red family presented a transmission rate of 0.343 (interval: 0.279 to 0.412), whereas that of the pRRL-GFP family was 0.484 (interval: 0.433 to 0.536). This suggests a delay in the integration process, as the embryos did not show any developmental delay. A third family issued from one founder generated with the pLVCTH vector presented the most important drop in the transmission rate, reaching 0.114 (interval: 0.773 to 0.161). As this latter family was derived from only one founder it was excluded from our study as a technical problem could possibly be the source of this difference. These different results raised a few questions.

Can differences among these vectors explain this large panel of transmission rates? As the zygote divides rapidly, a delay in any of the steps leading to integration will have an impact on the rate of transmission. During its journey from the plasma membrane to the cell nucleus, the lentiviral vector has to cope with important morphological and molecular changes. Lentiviral vectors enter the cell through the interaction of viral surface glycoproteins with receptors on the cell surface[33]. This binding causes a conformational change in the viral glycoproteins and fusion of the viral and cellular lipid bilayer, delivering the lentiviral RNA genome into the host cell. The viral genome then undergoes the reverse transcription, which is mediated by the viral retrotranscriptase brought in by the viral particle. The product of viral transcription is a blunt-ended double-stranded linear DNA, which is the substrate for viral integration within the nucleus. Any differences in vector size and/or secondary structures within the RNA genome could delay retrotranscription increasing thereby the time needed for integration. Secondary structures increase with the length of the DNA sequence. This could explain the difference between the small pRRL-GFP (around 7300bp) vector and pLV-tTRKRAB-red (around 11500bp). Moreover, the architecture of both vectors is different. Namely, pLV-tTRKRAB-red is a double cistronic vector tTRKRAB and dsRED coding sequences linked by an internal ribosomal entry site, known to form extensive secondary structures and thereby impinging on reverse transcription[168]. Thus, the length and the complexity of the vector construction could interfere with retrotranscription leading to a delay in integration and thereby to a genotypic mosaicism.

Ignoring technical considerations, the observation that the progeny containing the pLVCTH vector presents a very low transmission rate could be in part due to the complexity of its promoter region. pLVCTH contains a long chimeric promoter combining the human cytomegalovirus immediate-early enhancer and a modified chicken beta-actin promoter and first intron known to induce many secondary structures[169]. CAG promoter is among the most potent ubiquitous promoter used in lentiviral vectors.

Thus, according to our preliminary data, the choice of the promoter considering LVT should not only include its transcriptional robustness but also its complexity as any delay during the integration process can induce a strong genotypic mosaicism and a low transmission rate of the integrants to the progeny. However, from a practical point of view, a genetic mosaicism within transgenic animals generated by LVT is not of great importance as long as the animals contain more than one integrant. Whereas the transgenes integrate host DNA at only one locus following pronuclear injection, each lentivirus will separately integrate the DNA at different loci. Due to the weak level of lentiviral inactivation during embryogenesis, most proviruses will express the transgene. Thus, despite a genotypic heterogeneity, the transgenic animal will present a homogenous phenotype.

Another important factor that could alter the efficiency of integration is the viral titer. It is a well-known phenomenon that a lentiviral stock having a titer below 5×10^8 HeLa transducing unit/ml (HTU/ml) will barely produce transgenic animals. One reason could be that the embryo possesses restriction factors that will neutralize the incoming vector. However, as the transcriptional activity of a one-cell stage embryo is very low, these restriction factors have to be stored during the meiotic maturation of the oocyte and are thus in limited quantity. Therefore, the first lentiviral vectors to enter the cell could quench these restriction factors and free the way for the next one. This can explain why low titer vectors do not generate transgenic animals. The presence of host proteins that could inhibit the infection of vector may also explain why some species seem more resistant than others to lentiviral infection. It is now well established that species-specific host factors, called restriction factors, can alter the infectivity of retroviruses[170]. One such restriction factor, the tripartite motif protein TRIM5α, has recently emerged as an important restriction factor in mammals, blocking retroviral infection in a species-specific manner[171]. For example, Trim5α strongly inhibits retroviral infection in Monkeys, whereas its human counterpart is unable to restrict HIV infection, probably because human TRIM5α is not polymorphic in the regions B30.2 domain known to impact on viral recognition[172]. Whatever the molecular mechanism should be, the evolution of TRIM5α within the human genome probably impacts on HIV-1 transmission and/or pathogenesis in vivo. However, the anti-viral activity of TRIM5 orthologues in mammals other than primates remains poorly characterized[173]. A bovine TRIM (BoLv1) with broad antiretroviral activity suggests that TRIM-mediated restriction of retroviruses is widespread amongst mammals[174]. BoLv1 is closely related to TRIM5 genes suggesting that they are orthologues derived from an ancestral antiviral TRIM. The proof that a restriction factor inhibits within the murine embryo the retroviral infection following its perivitelline space injection should come from experiments showing a two hit kinetics. Different titers from the same batch of vector should reveal a threshold concentration above which any forthcoming vector integrates the genome of the embryo. The definitive proof for such a mechanism relies on the identification of the restriction factor, using for example co-immunoprecipitation techniques.

The presence or not of a restriction factor within the embryo with a species-specific expression and/or effect is very attractive but other more casualistic explanations can also be put forward to understand the relatively low transduction efficiency of lentiviral-mediated transgenesis. The volume of lentiviral vector injected into the perivitelline space can be roughly estimated as 10-100nl, knowing that it is strongly dependant on the quality of the vector and on the material used. Usually, a 0.5×10^9 HTU/ml or more viral stock is injected[101]. Thus, each embryo will be infected by around up to 10'000 viral particles. This number of particle by far exceed the usual dose used to transduce cell lines, where we can easily reach 100% of transduction with an multiplicity of infection ranging between 10 to 100. Interestingly, perivitelline space injection is not the sole technique to generate transgenic animals with lentiviral vectors. The zona pellucida can be removed with an acidic treatment and the denuded embryos can be infected with lentiviral vector. According to Lois et al., a concentration of 20×10^3 infectious units (IU)/µl were sufficient to get an average of 7 integrants per embryo, which is the average number of copy following the perivitelline injection of a 10^9 HTU/ml viral stock[101]. Thus considering that the diameter of an embryo is 80 µm, we can then calculate its volume and the number of viral particles in contact. Around 400 viral particles will surround the denuded embryo. This number is only a rough estimation, but this cannot explain the nearly 2 log difference between the co-culture experiment and the perivitelline injection to generate similar transgenic animals. Thus, the zona pellucida could act as an anti-viral barrier. In mammals, this membrane contains three to four sulphated glycoproteins called zona-pellucida protein-1 (ZP-1), ZP-2, ZP-3 and ZPB (in human only)[175]. These proteins are synthesized by and excreted from the oocyte during oogenesis and serves as primary and secondary sperm receptors as well as acrosome inducers. As these proteins are not known to display any antiviral activity, one explanation could be that the zona pellucida "glues" viral particles that are then unable to reach the plasmatic membrane.

Obviously, other explanations could be put forward to understand why such a high number of viral particles are needed to produce transgenic animals. For example, one could imagine that the reactivation of meiosis will impinge on the nuclear import of the pre-integration complex and redirected it toward degradation.

Whatever the mechanism, lentiviral transgenesis requires a highly concentrated vector[101]. Often, complicated vector designs will not produce good titers or the quality of the vector preparation will be too poor to be injected, then the infection of denuded embryos could be an alternative. This option is also economically interesting as there is no need for heavy material investment such as a station of injection. There are two major drawbacks however. First, the embryos without the zona pellucida cannot be transferred before the morula stage as they can be deleted by the oviductal musculature, and should therefore be kept in vitro. Moreover, they could implant ectopically within the oviductal wall creating life-threatening ectopic pregnancies. Second, following the removal of the zona pellucida, the embryos become very sticky and become difficult to manipulate decreasing the overall efficiency of the technique.

2.4.2 Integration site analysis

The genome-wide analysis of retroviral integration sites challenged our view on how these viruses pick up their landing spot in the target genome[84]. Briefly, retroviruses do not share the same strategy of integration. The two-best characterized retroviruses, MLV and HIV-1, present a bias for regions where they integrate into host genome. Thus, MLV will preferentially integrate near transcription start sites[84]. This characteristic can have an unfavourable impact on the transcriptional regulation of endogenous genes around the integration site. This scenario occurred during the first gene-therapy clinical trial that used MLV-based vectors to treat a rare genetic disease called X-linked severe combined immuno-deficiency disease (X-SCID)[176]. This disease is caused by the lack of a cytokine (Interleukine-7) receptor that leads to an early block in lymphocyte differentiation[177, 178]. The disrupted immune system is unable to mount any physiological responses against pathogens. This disease affects mostly children and leads to death within the first two years of life. Since 1968, the treatment of choice is allogenic bone marrow transplant that results in variable survival rates ranging from 46-97% depending on centers[179]. Until now, 14 children have been treated for X-SCID disease by gene therapy in UK and France. However, four of them developed leukaemia caused by insertions of MLV vector near the promoter region of the proto-oncogene LMO2[176]. The strong promoter contained within the MLV vector disrupted the physiological regulation of this endogenous gene, driving its overexpression.

Chapter 2. Genotypic features of lentiviral-derived transgenic mice

HIV-based lentiviral vectors present a different pattern of integration site[180]. They do not preferentially land near transcription start sites as MLV but tend to integrate within transcriptional units. Furthermore, the comparison of the integration sites within different cell types suggests that tissue-specific transcription results in tissue-specific biases in HIV integration site selection[84]. That is HIV-1 seems to target active genes. Thus, due to their differences in site-selection, the risk to activate endogenous genes by a read-through mechanism is a priori less important for HIV-based vectors than for their MLV-counterparts. Therefore, this observation puts HIV-based lentiviral vectors as an interesting alternative to MLV vectors for gene therapy. Moreover, as biosafety issues have been worked out with lentiviral vector design and production, the risk of recombinant competent retroviruses seems minimal if not inexistent[181].

In our study, we showed that in vivo lentiviral vectors recapitulate the in vitro pattern of integration. Using LAM PCR, we mapped 239 integration sites carried by 49 founders produced by lentiviral-mediated transgenesis. We observed that the integrations were significantly enriched in genes. A more refined analysis showed that, within genes, the integration tends to favour the middle of transcriptional units. Moreover, using LAM PCR methods, we were able to sequence individual integration sites and thus analyzed in details the different genes targeted by these vectors.

During the early preimplantation development, transposable elements (TE) are very active within the genome of the embryos. It has been suggested that they could play pivotal role in the expression or regulation of the early events governing the first days of life[182]. Repetitive elements encompass the different TEs that are found within the mouse genome, such as the long interspersed nuclear elements (LINE), the short interspersed nuclear elements (SINE) and the long terminal repeats elements[183]. In our transgenic mice, integrations into repeats were close to the fraction of repeats contained within the mouse genome (36% versus 38%, respectively). To determine whether this number was specific for transgenic mice, we transduced 3T3 fibroblasts with lentiviral vectors and analyzed the resulting integration sites. From the 108 integration sites mapped, only 24% were localized in repeats, contrasting with the 36% for the transgenic mice. This probably reflects the high activity of TE during the early preimplantation period and their inactivation later during the embryonic development[184, 185]. Their silencing is mainly due to epigenetic modifications, mostly methylation, that are completed at the blastocyst stage[186-188].

Interestingly, we found that 65% of the 239 integration sites were located within transcriptional units of unknown functions. To determine if lentiviral vectors could serve to detect transcriptional activity outside annotated genes, we designed exon-spanning primers based on GenScan predictions of the ENSEMBL database. Three out of 14 designs showed specific amplification profiles on genomic DNA. Next, considering the high percentage of lentiviral vectors integration into transcriptionally active units, we decided to analyze a few integration sites that were mapped into known genes to determine if their expression were higher during early development, corresponding to the time of integration. Interestingly, transcript levels of annotated lentiviral target genes were significantly higher in 2-cell embryos as compared to embryonic stem or adult cells, suggesting that these genes are more active during the early embryonic period and that they represent a more attractive target for lentiviral integration. Taken altogether, our data suggest that lentiviral vectors could "sense" transcriptional activity of a given cell type and integrate preferentially within these locations. As the pattern of integration among different lentiviruses, such as equine infectious anaemia virus (EIAV), feline immunodeficiency virus (FIV) or simian immunodeficiency virus (SIV), seems to be similar, this suggests that lentiviral vectors target an evolutionary conserved machinery to find their integration sites[189]. The lentiviral integrase protein could be one candidate. Namely, the integrase plays a pivotal role in site selection as the substitution of the HIV integrase for that of MLV cause the hybrid to integrate in a "MLV fashion"[85]. Moreover, it has been suggested that the lens-derived growth factor (LEDGF/p75), a cellular protein, could be an integrase partner implicated in the tethering of the preintegration complex within active region of host genome. LEDGF/p75 binds transcriptional units of the host genome and could act as a docking site for the incoming pre-integration complex through its interaction with the viral integrase[86].

We can only speculate why lentiviruses tend to integrate within transcriptional units whereas gammaretroviruses land in the vicinity of promoters. As discussed previously, one major difference between lentiviruses and gammaretroviruses is the capacity of the former to integrate the genome of non-dividing cells whereas the latter has to encounter a disorganized nuclear structure. Therefore, the strategy to integrate a compacted DNA structure has probably evolved to allow HIV to infect its target cells, the non-dividing T-cells and macrophages. During the past few years, progress has been made towards understanding the organization of the nucleus[190]. In differentiated nuclei, transcriptionally inactive "heterochromatin" is usually plastered against the inner face of the nuclear membrane. This heterochromatin is separated by nucleopores, shuttle channels between the cytoplasm and the nucleus, containing zones of active "euchromatin". Thus, in eukaryotic cells, we can differentiate between three classes of chromatin. The first form is the open or transcriptionally active chromatin containing genes with engaged RNA polymerases. The second is a form of repressed chromatin still prone to respond to activating signals. The third type accounts for most of the DNA in somatic cells and is composed of transcriptionally silent chromatin. Here genes are generally repressed in a heritable manner and promoters tend to be inaccessible for transcription factors. Interestingly, recent advances highlight the role of nuclear positioning in the control of gene expression[191, 192]. In this model, the nuclear-pore complexes (large multiprotein complexes (composed of about 30 proteins) that are embedded in the nuclear membrane and serves as gateways for traffic between nucleus and cytoplasm) play a pivotal role in the regulation of genes by coupling gene activation with its final RNA product[193, 194]. In this model, nuclear-pore complexes tether together the initiation complex and mRNA-processing complexes that are associated in the 3' UTR, inducing thereby a gene looping[195, 196]. This co-localization will help to fine-tune the expression of certain genes as the retention and/or the degradation of an aberrant mRNA near the site of transcription initiation can provide an immediate feed-back signal for the production of additional transcripts. Thus, the 5' and 3' ends of a gene together with the nuclear-pore complexes function as a checkpoint, having a global control on what gets in and what gets out of the transcriptional machinery. This complex molecular architecture will probably not facilitate the integration of an incoming pre-integration complex, whereas the gene loop seems to be a relatively accessible "landing spot". Therefore, the observation that lentiviruses tend to integrate within genes and not in the promoter regions could be due in part to the steric hindrance caused by those large proteinic complexes engaged in the transcriptional regulation and that the couple LEDG/p75 can only access and bind transcriptional units within the gene-loop, free of such large complexes. In our study, we observed an accumulation of lentiviral integrants in the middle of genes. This is in accordance with the gene-loop model as the tip of the loop should represent the middle of the gene and probably the most favourable area for integration. This model can also explain the observed bias of lentiviral integration within active genes, as those genes are more easily accessible than non-active ones embedded within the heterochromatin. In our study, 6 target genes out of a set of 8 were expressed at higher level in 2 cell stage embryos as compared to oocytes, suggesting that lentiviral vectors favoured genes transcriptionally active during early developmental stages. As lentiviral vectors integrate transcriptionally active regions of the genome, does it influence their activity? The lentiviral vector with its DNA cargo possesses all the molecular characteristics to affect the expression of its targeted gene. All the multiple steps leading to protein synthesis could be affected by the presence of a lentiviral vector. Our backcross experiments showed that only 8/104 animals could carry both copies of a same provirus within their genome. Thus, the presence of a provirus within a transcriptional unit tend to be deleterious to the overall survival rate, suggesting that lentiviral vectors once integrated can disrupt the expression of endogenous genes.

2.4.3 Limitations of lentiviral-mediated transgenesis

One major drawback of lentiviral vector use is the limited size of the DNA cargo (10Kb) they can carry between the LTRs. Sequences longer than 10Kb will interfere with the viral production, decreasing thereby the infectious titer. Therefore, alternative methods should be preferred when the transgene exceeds this cut-off value. Pronuclear injection allows the injection of large DNA sequence such as bacterial artificial chromosomes reaching up to 250Kb.[197] Other sequences such as polyA signals, recombination sites, or splicing sequences should be used cautiously in a lentiviral backbone as they can interfere with the normal processing of lentiviral vectors.

The success of the LVT is dependent on the quantity and the quality of the vector stock. Titers below 5×10^8 HeLa transducing unit rarely produce transgenic animals and the quality of the vector is a strong predictor of success as a poor quality preparation not only plugs the microcapillary but also increases the quantity of toxic molecules around the embryo, leading to premature embryonic death within minutes after the injection.

Usually, transgenic animals carry multiple integrants within their genome, making the establishment of pure inbred line difficult, as each provirus will segregate independently. Moreover, lentiviral vector can be more sensitive to epigenetic modifications than previously thought. A study performed in pigs showed that up to one third of integrants in the offspring was silenced or lowly expressed[103]. This lack of expression was probably linked to a high degree of methylation of CpG dinucleotides, as the administration of 5-azaC, a potent methylase inhibitor, was able to reactivate in vitro the expression of the transgene in the fibroblasts derived from the non-expressing animals. However, mechanism implying restriction factors, as discussed previously, cannot be rule out.

2.4.4 LAM and integration sites

Upon integration, lentiviral vector provides a DNA tag that can be used to map the integration site. Linear amplification PCR (LAM) was the technique used in our studies to retrieve the precise landing location into host genome[153]. Without entering into technical considerations, LAM PCR amplifies the junction between the provirus and the host neighbouring sequences. This stretch of DNA is then cloned into a plasmid and sequenced. These sequences are then annotated to the ENSEMBL mouse genome (version 41, http://www.ensembl.org/index.html). We then develop a convenient way to follow each individual integrant with the F1 and F2 generations. This was done by designing for each integration site three primers. One primer was specific for the LTR of lentiviruses and the two others were specific for the host genome flanking the provirus. For each integrant, two PCRs were performed: one that amplified the junction between the proviral LTR and the 3' host primer and the second that amplified the host region. This amplification is possible only if no provirus is lying between the 5' and 3' host primers, as the time allowed for amplification is not sufficient to cross the whole provirus.

The ISS PCR confirmed the presence of integrated lentiviral vectors within the sites mapped by LAM PCR. Transgenic animals are usually genotyped using pairs of primers that match the transgene. Then, the founder having the best profile of expression is kept to generate a transgenic line. As the pronuclear injection leads to transgene integration at one genetic locus, the progeny can be screened by the same PCR. If the pattern of expression differs in the progeny, a Southern blot analysis can be performed to determine whether integration occurred at other loci. However, the determination of the genetic status of animals produced by backcrosses can be more complicated. Backcrossing is a mandatory step to produce knockout animals or to obtain founders that transmit the transgene to all their progeny. In this situation, a PCR based on the transgene only will not discriminate between the homo- versus heterozygous status of the progeny. A semi-quantitative analysis can be performed by a Southern blot but this is not reproducible as it can often lead to false positive or negative. Usually, a more pragmatic approach is used to detect the founder that transmits the transgene to all its progeny by finding which one gives 100% of transmission. This technique is time consuming, as it will need enough pups to decrease the false positives, costly and ethically questionable, as it will engender the sacrifice of many animals. Thus, ISS PCR could be a rapid, simple and cost effective technique to determine the genetic status of the transgenic colony. Moreover, it will bring some additional information on the integration site that could help to choose the best fitted founder. This could for example decrease the ectopic expression of the transgene (positional effects) that can be observed when the integration takes place in the vicinity of genes or enhancer regions. Moreover, integration within genes that can lead to gene inactivation or hypomorphic alleles could be discarded, providing that the landing site is known.

Chapter 3
Study of lineage commitment of early blastomeres

3.1 Introduction

The cell fate decisions that govern the earliest steps of mammalian embryonic development are still poorly understood [198]. In particular, the stage at which early blastomeres become committed either to the inner cell mass (ICM), which subsequently yields the embryo proper, or to the trophectoderm, which is the precursor of extra-embryonic tissues, is a matter of debate [4]. The long held "random" hypothesis for development of the embryonic-abembryonic axis states that, within these two structures, early blastomeres are equally represented [4, 199, 200]. However, recent lineage-tracing experiments support to a model of "developmental bias", in which the progeny of the early blastomeres is allocated in a biased fashion [5, 117]. For instance, it was found that, whilst both blastomeres of a 2-cell stage embryo participate in giving rise to the ICM and the trophectoderm, one cell contributes predominantly to the embryonic part of the blastocyst –the site of the polar trophectoderm and ICM- and the other to the abembryonic part –the site of the mural trophectoderm and more superficial ICM cells- [125]. Furthermore, when blastomeres separated at the 4-cell stage were pooled according to position and implanted into foster mothers, only those issued from the "animal" pole could yield embryos, suggesting early differences in the developmental capacity of individual blastomeres [126]. Interestingly, Fujimori et al. followed the progeny of blastomeres beyond the blastocyst stage using the Cre-lox system[201]. They used transgenic blastomeres that expressed LacZ only upon injection of a Cre plasmid within their nucleus. They could therefore specifically tag a blastomere and study its contribution to the developing embryo by performing a LacZ staining. Their data showed that the derivatives of one blastomere tagged at the two cell stage randomly mixed with cells originating from the second blastomere in the different layers examined, suggesting that they contributed equally and randomly to the ICM and trophectoderm. However, a labelling at the 4-cell stage presented a different picture, as the tagged blastomere showed preferentially a localized contribution to either the trophectoderm or ICM, although some mixed contributions were also noticed.

Chapter 3. Study of lineage commitment of early blatomeres

A few years later, the same group used a new non-invasive technique to study the contribution of the 2-cell stage blastomeres during the pre-implantation development[202]. To do so, they established a transgenic mouse strain that ubiquitously expresses a fluorescent protein that emits green fluorescence that can be turned to red after exposure to weak ultraviolet. After the selective exposition of one of both blastomeres to UV, they were transferred to a surrogate mother till the blastocyst stage. They observed no tendency of one or the other blastomeres to contribute either to the embryonic or abembryonic regions of the blastocyst. Interestingly, they showed that when the movement of the embryo within the zona pellucida is restricted-which is mainly the case during in vitro experiments- a correlation between cell lineage and the axis of the blastomere can be observed. In other words, the observed bias in lineage observed in certain studies could in part be explained by their experimental settings, impinging the embryo to move freely within the zona pellucida. This study not only pointed out the great capacity of the developing embryos to adapt to exogenous cues but also that any attempts to study the early embryonic development should be performed as physiological as possible to minimize experimental bias. Therefore, we decided to study the lineage commitment of early blastomeres retrospectively, analyzing tissues derived from embryos at E12.5 previously transduced with lentiviral vectors at the one- or two-cell stage. As lentiviral integrations are independent from each other, creating a molecular signature, they can be used to differentiate the progeny of two cells independently transduced. As our previous study suggested that the kinetic of integration in murine embryo is a rapid event occurring between the one-or two-cell stages, we examined the lineage commitment of early blastomeres, using lentivirus integration sites as molecular lineage tracing tags[203]. Our results suggest that, in a majority of cases, these cells are assigned to either the inner cell mass or the trophectoderm shortly after the first cell division, in agreement with a view whereby lineage commitment is biased early on.

Chapter 3. Study of lineage commitment of early blatomeres

3.2 Material and methods

3.2.1 Lentiviral-mediated transgenesis

We generated transgenic mice by perivitelline injection of fertilized oocytes, as described[101]. Briefly, the hybrid strain B6D2G1 derived from C57BL/6JxDBA2J (Charles River Company) was used as egg donor. Superovulation was induced by intra-peritoneal (IP) injection of five B6D2G1 female with 10 IU of Pregnant Mare Serum (PMS) (Sigma). Forty-six hours later, a second IP injection was performed with 10 IU of Human Chorionic Gonadotropin (HCG) (Sigma), before mating with B6D2G1 males. Sixteen hours later, oocytes were harvested, injected in the perivitelline space with a highly concentrated vector stock (5×10^8-1×10^9 HeLa transducing unit/ml), and kept in culture overnight at 37°C and 5% CO_2 in KSOM medium (Specialty Media). Embryos that had reached the 2-cells stage were then placed in the ampulla of foster NMRI mothers (8 embryos per ampulla). All vectors used in this study were previously described [70]. Genotyping of the offspring was done by PCR using vector-specific primers (forward primer: 5'-TATGTTGCTCCTTTTACGCTATGTG-3, reverse primer: 5'-CGACAACACCACGGAATTGT-3').

3.2.2 Southern blot

One-cell stage embryos were collected from B6D2G1 females and were randomly separated in two pools: the first was immediately injected with concentrated pRRL-GFP (6×10^8 HeLa transducing unit/ml) as described above, the second kept in culture until the first division before vector injection. After overnight incubation, each set of embryos was implanted into the ampulla of pseudopregnant NMRI females. At E12.5 days later, conceptuses were harvested and embryos separated from placenta by dissection. DNA was purified from both tissues by overnight digestion in lysis buffer, phenol-chloroform extraction and ethanol precipitation. 5µg of DNA was digested with PvuII, separated on 0.8% agarose gel in TBE buffer, transferred to Hybond+ nylon membranes (Amersham, USA) and hybridized (Church buffer: 50 ml NaPi 1M, 35 ml SDS 20%, 15 ml H_2O, 0.2 ml EDTA 0.5M) with a DIG-labelled probe specific for WPRE amplified by PCR (forward primer: 5'-TATGTTGCTCCTTTTACGCTATGTG-3, reverse primer: 5'-CGACAACACCACGGAATTGT-3') (PCR DIG labelling mix, Roche Applied Science).

3.3 Results

3.3.1 Lentivectors to analyse blastomeric fate

We injected lentiviral vectors into the perivitelline space of either one- or two-cell stage embryos and transplanted these to pseudo-pregnant females. We then harvested the resulting conceptuses at E12.5, separated embryos from placentas by dissection, and compared the patterns of proviral integration in these two tissues by Southern blotting (Fig. 9A). From five conceptuses infected at the one-cell stage, we obtained 59 integrations, 28 in embryos and 31 in placenta. Twenty-five of the placental integrants were also present in the corresponding embryos. Therefore, after infection of 1-cell embryos, 73% of the insertions were shared between placenta and embryo, whereas 27% were found either in placenta (18%) or in the embryo (9%) exclusively. In contrast, among 233 proviruses present in 27 conceptuses resulting from infections at the two-cell stage, only 42 (22%) were common to both embryonic and extra-embryonic tissues (Fig. 9B).

Chapter 3. Study of lineage commitment of early blatomeres

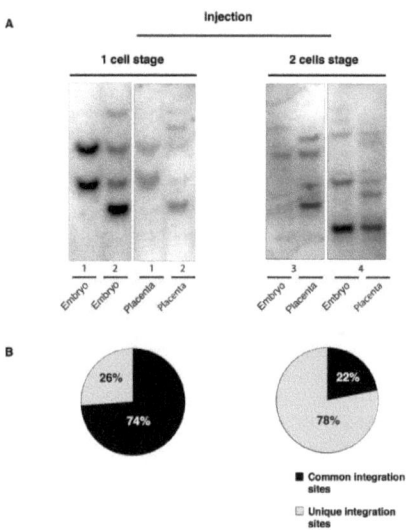

Fig. 9. Embryonic vs. abembryonic distribution of proviruses as a function of time of infection
(A) Southern blot analysis of the proviruses found in placenta or embryonic body of conceptuses (1 to 4) injected at one-cell (left) or two-cell (right) stages. (B) Cumulative results of the analysis of 59 (left panel) and 233 (right panel) proviruses present in embryos injected at the one- and two-cell stage, respectively. Intervals of confidence (95%) were 0.129-0.444 for one-cell stage injections and 0.715-0.837 for two-cell stage injections. P<0.0001 (Fischer's exact test).

3. 4 Conclusion

The mammalian embryo has around five days to reach the blastocyst stage and to build the first morphological differences, notably to form the inner cell mass (ICM) and the trophectoderm[110]. During this period, the blastomeres are considered to be identically totipotent, allowing each of them to generate an entire organism. Moreover, they present a remarkable plasticity as the loss of one blastomere is not deleterious for the ongoing development and is compensated by the other cells. Interestingly, in other organisms such as Drosophila melanogaster, Xenopus laevi or C.elegans the establishment of the body axes is already set up at the one cell stage[115, 116]. During oogenesis, different morphogenetic determinants are unevenly distributed within the cytoplasm, creating, upon fertilization, morphogenic gradients that will specifically contribute to the building of the body axis. Thus, the loss of one cell or even the loss of part of the cytoplasm of the oocyte will considerably impair normal development[119, 120].

In mammals, embryonic polarity is a later event and is established during the first days of development, with the definition of three major axes (dorsoventral, head-tail and left-right)[204]. Whether blastomeres issued from the first cell divisions establish this polarity as a result of early set differences biasing their fate or, alternatively, whether such fates are determined significantly later as the result of cell-to-cell interactions[205] remains to be fully understood. A long held assumption was that, until the blastocyst stage and the first apparition of morphological differences with the development of the embryonic and extra-embryonic poles, cells forming the early embryos are randomly assigned to these structures, independently of previous events[200, 206]. An emerging model states that early embryos show a developmental bias in that, for most of them, the progeny of one of the two primitive blastomeres gives rise to either the embryonic, or the extra-embryonic part of the blastocyst[5]. In this view, the preferential allocation of blastomeres to either the embryonic or abembryonic tissues depends on the order and orientation of the second cleavage of the mouse embryo[4, 126]. Accordingly, lineage-tracing experiments using injected dyes and beads and transfer of individual blastomeres to donor embryos showed that blastomeres at the four-cell stage differ in their developmental success and properties[126]. Most recently, it has been suggested that epigenetic modifications could be the underlying mechanism influencing cell fate determination[207].

Chapter 3. Study of lineage commitment of early blatomeres

We used lentiviral vectors as tags to examine the lineage commitment of early blastomeres. While infection of fertilized oocytes with these vectors yielded integrants subsequently found for their majority in both embryonic and extra-embryonic tissue, infection of two-cell stage embryos induced a drastically different picture, with only a minority of integrants shared between both types of tissues. In our protocol, the first cleavage occurs normally about 12 hours after the injection of the 1-cell embryos (data not shown). A PCR-based analysis of the kinetics of lentivirus/HIV integration revealed that, in human T lymphoid cells, integration starts 4h after infection and reaches its maximum after 16h corroborating our published data suggesting that lentiviral integration occurs rapidly in the embryo and supporting the idea that lentiviruses can be efficiently used as tags for cell-lineage tracing experiments[162,203]. This approach is less invasive than those based on the injection of a dye or of a CRE recombinase-expressing plasmid [201], since the lentivector is injected in the perivitelline space and not in the embryo itself. The genomic tag provided by the integrated provirus is stable, and provides means to follow the fate of individual blastomeres.

The observation of proviral integrations specific to the embryonic or abembryonic lineage indicates that early blastomeres are contributing differentially to these lineages and argues against a purely stochastic model. However, we still obtained 22% of shared integrations after infection at the 2-cell stage, with only 8 out of 27 embryos showing a complete segregation of the provirus integration patterns, implying that a fully "determined" model does not reflect the reality either. Therefore, our observations rather support the "developmental bias" hypothesis [121]. Furthermore, the sharp drop in the percentage of shared insertion events when the injection was performed at the two-cell stage (likely corresponding to integration occurring at this or the four-cell stage) implies that the commitment of individual blastomeres occurs at around the time of the second cleavage. This corroborates previous evidence demonstrating that blastomeres from the 4-cell stage on tend to have a reduced developmental potential, suggesting that they are already committed to a specific fate [126]. Interestingly, Zernicka-Goetz [125] and Fujimori and colleagues [201] observed that for about 70% of the embryos, the progeny of single blastomeres where mostly allocated to one region of the blastocysts. Our study substantiates these observations and thus gives further support to an early bias model for the developmental fate of two- to four-cell stage blastomeres. In addition, our comparative analyses of embryonic and placental DNAs revealed not only distinct proviral integration patterns for the two tissues, notably after infection of two-cell stage embryos, but also an apparently higher degree of heterogeneity in the intensity of the bands detected by Southern blot in the placenta. Although this result would have to be verified using a larger number of samples, it nonetheless suggests that the placenta exhibits a greater level of mosaicism than the embryo, that is, is derived from a greater fraction of the early blastomeres.

3.4.1 Benefits and limitations

The design of our study relied on the presence or absence of a signature -the lentiviral vector- within tissues derived from the ICM or the trophectoderm, contrasting in that with the vast majority of studies devoted to clarify the fate of the early blastomeres. Namely, the retrospective analysis of confocal images of tagged blastomeres and its inherent in-vitro setting is often subject to controversy, stemming from the difficulty in delineating the physical boundaries between the embryonic and abembryonic parts of the embryo. This is an important point, as different limits will directly impact on the percentage of blastomeres contributing to the ICM or not. Moreover as embryonic development is an active process, the limits between these two structures cannot be fixed without increasing false positive or negative in the statistical analysis. In our analysis, we do not rely on arbitrarily boundaries but on end products, limiting thereby the risk of misinterpretation. Of note, the question of the mouse strain was raised as a possible explanation for the discrepancies observed among the different studies[4]. Here, we used the same F2 embryos derived from the mating of two hybrid B6D2F1 (C57BL/6J xDBA/2J) that were used in the Alarcon and Marikawa's study, where they showed no bias in blastomeric fate[7].

Our study presents further advantages. First, our embryos were collected and analyzed at D12.5, contrasting with the blastocyst stage of all the different studies performed in this field with the exception of the Fujimori's study[201]. Second, our embryos remained only one day and a half in culture as compared to the 4.5-5 days for the other studies and were transferred in utero for the rest of their development. Third, the integrity of the embryo was preserved, as we did not cross the plasma membrane. Finally, as we used the same batch of vector to generate our transgenic mice, no difference inherent to the vector stock quality can be put forward.

As the number of integration sites analyzed in our study was low and only a limited number of outlying animals could have a strong impact on the statistic, we reanalyzed our data by eliminating one by one every animal from the statistic to observe if a discrepancy occurred. This was not the case and the statistic remained the same (data not shown). Another criticism could be the sensitivity of our Southern blot analysis. Considering that all blastomeres contributed to both embryonic and abembryonic structures but at different degree, one could argue that the mosaicism is such that the number of certain integrants are too low to be detectable. We used a Southern blot protocol using DIG-labelled probe that could detect a single copy gene according to the manufacturer (Roche diagnostics, AG). Nevertheless, as efficient as this technique could be, if the contribution of one blastomere within the placenta is very low, we would not have been able to detect it. Another argument against drawing conclusions from our results could be the contamination of the placental DNA with that of the yolk sac. This structure derives from the primitive endoderm which itself derived from the ICM. Therefore, these two structures are genotypically identical and the yolk sac is often used to genotype the embryo. The yolk sac is closely apposed to the placenta and has to be removed carefully before cutting a piece of placenta. If this procedure is not made properly, it could lead to the contamination of placental DNA with embryonic DNA. But what could have been the implication of this DNA contamination on our results? For the pool of conceptuses derived from one-cell stage injection, not much. For the other pool it would have increased the number of common sites between the placenta and the embryo. The percentage of common sites would have increased in parallel. As the difference in common versus unique sites was important in our results, it suggested that our dissection were careful.

Nevertheless, our study has some limitations. As already mentioned, the number of integration sites analyzed is too low- even if the data seem significant- to draw any hard conclusions. A few questions remain to be clarified. For example, Kurotaki et al showed that blastomeres that were not moving freely within the zona pellucida could present a false lineage bias[202]. Thus, as the lentiviral preparation is very viscous, its presence within the perivitelline space could glue the embryo, altering thereby its rotation and inducing an experimental bias toward lineage specification. Our experimental setting implied an in vitro culture of our embryos during 72 hours, allowing time for the lentiviruses to transduce them. This experimental setting could further alter the rotation of our embryos. Moreover, as the chemical tags used in different studies or the fluorescent microscopy could have altered the embryonic development, the different procedures used during the perivitelline injection such as the squeezing of the embryo or the inherent toxicity of the vector preparations could have disrupted the physiology of development. Our previous study showed that lentiviral vectors integrate rapidly into the fertilized oocyte once injected within the perivitelline space. However, the time needed to integrate a 2-cell stage embryo is not known, although we speculated that the kinetic was similar in both cases. The activation of the embryonic genome, the rapid divisions of the initial blastomeres and the maternal RNA degradation could all have a negative impact on the incoming vector, creating a delay in its integration. Thus, the strong shift in integration pattern that we observed could be due to a postponed integration of the vectors and not to intrinsic differences between the blastomeres. This would be in accordance with published data showing that from the 4-cell stage on, differences in blastomere allocation exist[201,125]. One interesting experiment could be to freeze transiently the embryonic divisions at the time of transduction and to perform the same analysis. The repetition of our results will then favour the model of an intrinsic difference between the blastomeres. Other experiments could be designed to speed up the integration at the two-cell stage. For example, the fertilized oocyte could be injected using a temperature-sensitive integrase and allowed to perform its first division at restrictive temperature. Once the two-cell stage is reached, the embryo could be grown at a permissive temperature, allowing the integration of the vector. As the PIC should already be located within the nucleus, it should integrate the host genome faster than a lentivector injected within the perivitelline space at that embryonic stage.

If embryos showed a bias toward one cell type, a molecular explanation would have to be found for this differential fate. Only one recent study proposed a molecular mechanism for the developmental bias model[207]. It showed that 4-cell stage blastomeres present different degree of epigenetic modifications according to their future contribution to either the ICM or trophectoderm. The authors also observed that the level of methylation of the histone H3 at specific arginine residues is maximal in blastomeres that will contribute to the ICM, whereas arginine methylation is only minimal in cells whose progeny contribute more to trophectoderm. Moreover, by overexpressing Carm1, which specifically methylates H3, in individual blastomeres they were able to direct the progeny of these cells to the ICM. A molecular analysis showed an upregulation of known stem cell-specific transcription factors such as nanog and sox-2[208, 209]. These results are appealing as stem cells are directly derived from the ICM and emerging concepts point to epigenetic modifications as probable key players in the maintenance of stemness. Namely, ES cells seem to be characterized by a distinct higher-order global chromatin structure. Studies in several systems indicate that ES cells are richer in less compact euchromatin and, as differentiation progresses, accumulate highly condense, transcriptionally inactive heterochromatin regions[188]. In this model, epigenetic modifications play a role of gatekeeper that open or close the access of transcription factors to chromatin, notably through the action of histone methylases[210].

Nevertheless, considering the very early stage -probably before the 4-cell stage according to our experiment- at which a fate-decision is made, the idea that maternally-derived information might impact to different degrees in individual blastomeres is appealing. As previously noted, non-mammalians development is governed by morphogenic determinants embedded within the cytoplasm, but such determinants have never been found in mammals. Still, the recent discovery that small non-coding RNAs could impact on a variety of biological process through post-transcriptional modulation of gene expression changed our traditional view on the role of the RNA family and on gene expression[72]. In particular, miRNAs are a class of short (19-25 nucleotides), single stranded RNAs that are present in plants and animals. Interestingly, in vitro experiments have shown that over expression of a single miRNAs can decrease the level of more than 100 mRNAs. This observation has led to the hypothesis that miRNAs could act as developmental switches or, more subtly, to sharpen the border of spatial or temporal gene-expression domains. The global function of miRNAs in development can be inferred from animals that lack of DICER 1, a cytoplasmic RNase III involved in miRNA maturation. Such deletions result in mice in an early developmental arrest, accompanied by defects in the proliferation of pluripotent stem cells[211]. It is yet well established that, later in development, miRNAs play pivotal roles in the numerous cells such as neurones, myocytes and lymphocytes[212]. Therefore, future lines of research should focus on differential miRNAs patterns between early blastomeres as a potential source of fate determination.

3.4.2 The prepatterning vs. regulative model

Our data and evidence from other laboratories suggest that the two initial blastomeres tend to follow distinct developmental paths. But on the other hand, we know that if we had separated these two blastomeres, they had the intrinsic potentiality to support the development of two entire organisms. How then can we put together these two a priori contradictory lines of evidence? One possible mechanism is that a morphogenic gradient exists in the egg or the embryo, and that it relies on the relative and not the absolute concentration of an effector (miRNA?). This supposes that when the polarity is disturbed, the gradient is not lost and can be sufficient to direct proper development. Another idea could be that cell-cell interaction actively repress or activate pathways that drive differentiation and whenever this arrangement is disturb, it will reactivate a default pathways that will rebuild the asymmetric differentiation. The central idea here is that it is not totipotency which represents the default state of blastomeres but programmed differentiation. The Par3/aPKC complex can be an interesting candidate, as it is known to have a role in establishing the polarity in different organisms[213]. Interestingly, this complex adopts a polarized localization on mouse embryo as soon as the 8-cell stage. Moreover, the downregulation of Par3 or the injection of a dominant negative form of aPKC positioned the progeny of the manipulated blastomere inside the embryo, leading to an increase tendency to form ICM cells[214].

Chapter 4
Development of a new lentiviral gene trap vector

4.1 Introduction

As our in vivo results confirmed in vitro experiments showing that lentiviral vectors integrate preferentially into transcriptionally active regions of the genome, we exploited this feature to design a new kind of gene trap vector. When lentiviral vectors infect a fertilized oocyte, integration of the vector DNA occurs before or at the two-cell stage. Based on the demonstrated trend of Lentiviral vectors to hit active transcriptional units, integration should be enhances into genes active during the preimplantation period. Recent large-scale transcriptome analysis have shed some light on critical events of this developmental period[128], revealing that genes specifically transcribed within the preimplantation embryo present a pattern of transient wave-like activation, during and following the degradation of maternally derived transcripts. However, such studies are limited to the probes spotted on the microarray and do not probe genomic loci with yet unknown function. Thus, we wondered if lentiviral vectors could be used as a tool to hit and manipulate active transcriptional units of the developing mouse. Our studies had demonstrated that lentiviral vectors favour transcriptional units expressed at higher level in early blastomeres as compared to embryonic stem cells or differentiated cell lines such as 3T3 fibroblasts[203]. Moreover, we showed that G2 animals issued from the backcross of the founder with its progeny led to a decreased percentage of living animals, suggesting that essential genes were inactivated by bi-allelic proviral integration. Therefore, we decided to construct a lentiviral gene trap vector to capture and study genes expressed in the early embryonic period.

4.2 Material and methods

4.2.1 Lentiviral trap vector

Briefly, we subcloned the different components in a pUC18 vector (Fermentas International). Five µg of pUC 18 plasmid was digested for 2h at 37°C in 50µl solution containing 5µl NEB Buffer 2 (New England Biolab) and 2U HindIII and 2U AflIII (New England Biolab). The digestion was loaded on 0.8% Agarose gel and run for 45 min at 80V. The linearized vector was purified using a Qiagen gel extraction kit following instruction (Qiagen, cat N°; 28706). 5 µg of this plasmid was linked to a linker (5' agcttggg atttaaat tggcca ggcgcgcc tccgga gtcgac atcgat accggt atttaaatt 3', Microsynth, Switzerland)in a 20µl solution containing 2µl NEB ligase buffer (New England Biolab) and 2µl of Ligase (New England Biolab, CatN°M0202L) for 10 min at RT. The solution was purified using PCR purification kit (Qiagen). Next, we performed different PCR reactions on the published vector pRRL.SIN.cPPT.PGK.GFP[215].The PCR reaction started with an initial activation step of 95°C for 15 min (Hotstart), followed by 10 cycles of 94°C 45'', 60°C (-1°C per cycle) for 45'', 72°C for 1' (touchdown), and 30 cycles of 94°C for 45'', 50°C for 45'', 72°C for 1' and a final extension at 72°C for 10'. The PCR reactions were the purified using PCR kit (Qiagen), resuspended in 30 µl of Tris-EDTA.

The primers used are found within the following table:

Oligo	Seq (5'-3')/Sense primer	Oligo	Seq (5'-3')/anti-sense primer
Intron For	atcaagcttatcgataccgtc	Intron Rev	gaaccggtgaagttcctatactttctaga gaataggaacttcggaataggaacttcg taccgagctcgaattgatc
PolyA For	taggtcgacgccgccaccatggcaataa cttcgtatagcatacattatacgaagttata catgttcgactagtgggtttaaacccgcct cgactgtgccttctag	PolyA Rev	agctccggaataacttcgtataggatact ttatacgaagttatcctggtaccaggatc gagccccagctggtt
IRES For	cggtatcataagcttgattaagtagctgata cgcgtcgacaagcttgattaa gtagctgat	IRES Rev	ctcggccatggttaagctaattcgatg

Chapter 4. Development of a new lentiviral gene trap vector

The PCR products were cloned using standard procedure. Briefly, a 30μl solution containing 3μl of specific NEB buffer matching the restriction enzymes used for 2 hours at 37°C (please refer to the NEB chart for RE buffer). Then, the digestion was loaded on 0.8% Agarose gel and run for 45 min at 80V. The PCR product was purified using a Qiagen gel extraction kit following instruction (Qiagen, cat N°; 28706) and then ligated to the polylinker found within the pUC18 in a 20μl solution containing 2μl NEB ligase buffer (New England Biolab) and 2μl of Ligase (New England Biolab, CatN°M0202L) for 10 min at RT. The solution was purified using PCR purification kit (Qiagen). The different digestions were performed as follow: Intron: AgeI-ClaI, PolyA: BspEi-SalI and IRES:ClaI-NcoI. Finally, the LacZ sequence was extracted from the pLacZ (gift from F.Spitz). Five μg of pLacZ and 5μg of the pUC18 were independently digested for 2h at 37°C in 50μl solution containing 5μl NEB Buffer 2 (New England Biolab) and 2U NcoI and 2U SpeI (New England Biolab). The digestions were loaded on 0.8% Agarose gel and run for 45 min at 80V. The linearized vector and the DNA sequence were purified using a Qiagen gel extraction kit following instruction (Qiagen). 5 μl of each eluate were ligated in a 20μl solution containing 2μl NEB ligase buffer (New England Biolab) and 2μl of Ligase (New England Biolab, CatN°M0202L) for 10 min at RT. The solution was purified using PCR purification kit (Qiagen). Finally, the gene trap construction was cloned within the lentiviral backbone pRRL-GFP.

4.2.2 ES cells culture

ES cells E14 (gift from D.Duboule) were grown in DMEM for ES cells (Specialty Media) supplemented with 15% heat-inactivated FCS, 1,000 units of leukemia inhibitory factor/ml (Gibco), and the following reagents (Specialty Media): 1% penicillin-streptomycin, 1% l-glutamine, 1% nonessential amino acids, 1% nucleosides, and 1% β-mercaptoethanol. Cells were split 1:3 or 1:4 every 24 h. Cells were cultured in feeder-free conditions on gelatin 0.1% coated plates.

The ES cells were transduced in suspension with our gene trap vector at a MOI 30 following their splitting. 6 hours later, the ES cells were washed with PBS and fresh medium were added.

4.2.3 LacZ staining

The ES cells in 12 well plates were washed once with PBS and fixed for 10 minutes using a solution containing PBS 1%PFA, 0.2% Glutaraldehyde. Then, after a second wash with PBS, the staining solution (A 1ml LacZ staining solution contain 960µl PBS (Sigma), 20µg $MgCl_2$(1M), 20µl of 0.2M Potassium Ferricyanide (Sigma), 20µl of 0.2M Potassium Ferrocyanide and 10µl X-Gal (Invitrogen, CatN°:15520018) was added to the cells and put back at 37°C overnight.

4.3 Results and discussion

4.3.1 Overview

In this gene trap vector, translation of the endogenous gene stops upon splicing at one of three tandem stop codons inserted in every reading frame. Successful trapping can be followed by de novo translation of the reporter gene initiated in a cap-independent manner from the mouse encephalomyocarditis virus internal ribosomal entry site (IRES)[216]. We replaced the marker gene by lacZ flanked by heterologous lox sites allowing cassette exchange and inserted two inverted FRT sites spanning the entire trapping cassette[217]. In case the vector is integrated in antisense to the transcriptional orientation of the target gene, FLIP can be used to change the orientation of the vector cassette (Fig.10A). To determine the functionality of the vector, we transduced murine ES cells at low multiplicity of infection (MOI). We isolated 168 ES clones after limiting dilution, lentiviral vector-specific sequences could be detected in 56 out of 168 (33.3%) clones. To calculate the trapping efficiency of our lentiviral trapping vector, we stained 48 vector-positive clones with b-Gal. Figure 10B shows 3 lacZ positive ES-cell clones representing the varying expression levels detected. In total 7 out of 48 clones stained blue (14.6%). These data suggested that our lentiviral trapping vector successfully trapped endogenous genes expressed in murine ES cells.

Chapter 4. Development of a new lentiviral gene trap vector

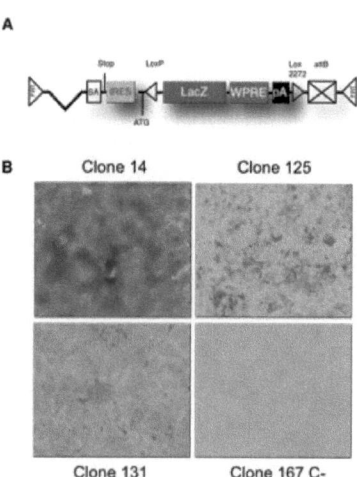

Fig. 10. A Schematic representation of the lentiviral gene trap vector. This vector contains two main modules: one contained within the FRT sites and allowing the switch of the whole vector in the correct transcriptional orientation and a second one encompassing the expression cDNA and allowing its exchange when needed. Of note, a stop codon in all three reading frame aborts endogenous translation to favour the new initiation of translation contained with the IRES leading to the in-frame translation of the reporter gene. Finally, an attB site in the 3' end could be used to insert a new cDNA, once the vector is already integrated. B. Four different ES clones are shown with different LacZ expression reflecting the potency of the trapped genes.

To test whether the lacZ expression cassette can be inverted, we analyzed lacZ-negative ES colonies for the presence of lentiviral vector sequences. We isolated 45 PCR positive but lacZ negative ES clones suggesting that the reporter gene was either not functional or integrated in antisense to the endogenous transcriptional unit. Upon transfection of a FLIP-expressing plasmid, we could detect lacZ expression in two ES cell clones. A PCR

Chapter 4. Development of a new lentiviral gene trap vector

confirmed the new orientation of the trapping vector (not shown) (Figure 11).

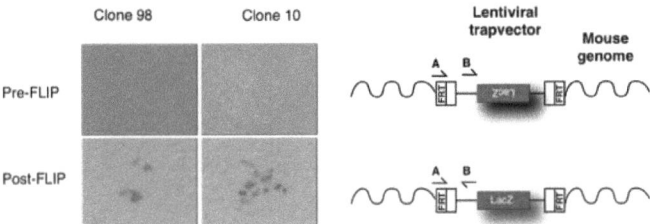

Fig. 11. The use of the FRT site can rescue the expression of a trapping vector. The upper left panel shows two ES clones containing a trapping vector in the false transcriptional orientation (Clone 98 and 10 Pre-FLIP). The upper right panel schematically represents the genetic situation. Upon electroporation of a Flipase plasmid, some ES cells will express the transgene (lower left), consistent with the reorientation of the cDNA. The lower right panel depicts the new genetic situation.

Next, we tested whether the lacZ expression cassette could be exchanged in vitro. We transfected lacZ positive ES cells with both a Cre-expressing plasmid and a donor plasmid containing the hygromycin-GFP reporter gene, surrounded by donor lox sites (Figure 12A). Three weeks after hygromycin selection, one ES-cell clone expressed GFP at two distinct levels (Figure 12C). To exclude GFP-expression from episomal, non-integrated forms of the

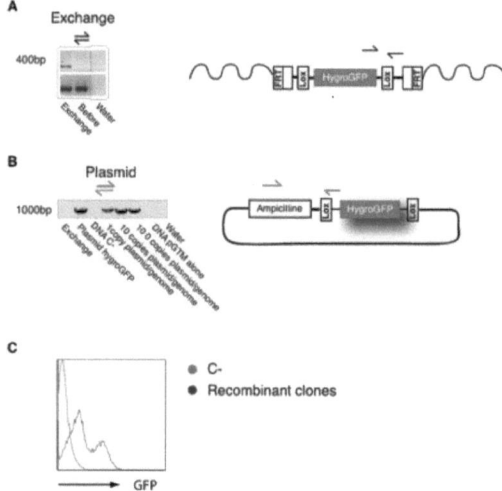

Fig. 12. cDNA exchange between plasmid and integrated trapping vector. A. Left. PCR analysis of a successful exchange between LacZ expressing ES cells before and after exchange. Right. The primers were chosen to amplify only the integrated Hygro-GFP. The genetic situation after the exchange LacZ-Hygro-GFP is also depicted B. Left. PCR amplification showing no plasmid contamination within our recombinant ES cells. Right. Primers position on plasmid. C. FACS analysis of ES clone showing eGFP expression at two different levels after cassette exchange.

donor plasmid we screened by PCR for the presence of the bacterial selection marker ampicillin. We detected the non-integrated donor plasmid as low as one copy per genome whereas no such PCR signal was detectable in this ES-cell clone suggesting that the non-integrated plasmid had been diluted out during cell growth (Fig. 12B). Using a different PCR targeting a sequence in the integrated vector (attB) and GFP derived from the donor plasmid, we

Chapter 4. Development of a new lentiviral gene trap vector

demonstrated successful cassette exchange in this ES-cell clone. Taken together these data suggested successful trapping of genes endogenously expressed in murine ES cells and that the provirus could be further manipulated improving thereby its functionality.

4.3.2 Experimental perspectives for a lentiviral gene trap vector

Having this lentiviral vector at hand, different applications can be envisioned. First, this gene trap vector can be an interesting tool to use vitro. Namely, gene trapping was developed as a high-through put alternative to the time-consuming and costly gene targeting strategies and were mainly performed on embryonic stem (ES) cells[218, 219].

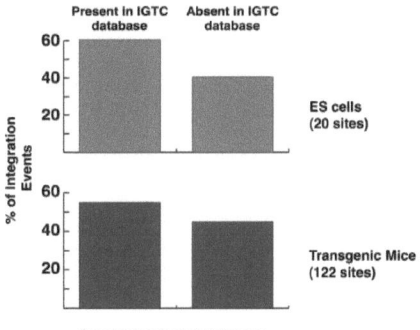

Fig. 13. Comparison of the integration profile between the lentiviral gene trap vectors in ES cell and in vivo and the international gene trap consortium database. These diagrams show that the lentiviral gen trap vector could be complementary to the other strategies to trap the entire genome.

Chapter 4. Development of a new lentiviral gene trap vector

To date only MLV- or plasmid-based gene trap vectors were used in an attempt to cover the entire transcriptome of the murine genome[220]. These high throughput experiments lead to the mutation of nearly two thirds of the mouse genome. However, gene trapping is not linear and decreases after ca 100'000 insertions to a rate of one new gene discovered for 35 insertions. Lentiviral gene trap vectors could therefore be a complementary strategy to saturate the entire mouse genome with trapped transcriptional units (fig.13). Second, as we showed that lentiviral vectors present an integration bias for active transcriptional units in the transgenic mouse, we could combine the power of gene trap design to transgenesis to get access to new genes active during preimplantation development. The general strategy would be to generate transgenic males carrying low copy numbers of lentiviral gene trap vectors. Then, we could analyze the integration sites of the lentiviral vectors within each founder by LAM PCR. These males could then be mated with wild-type females and the resulting embryos could be analyzed for their pattern of LacZ expression. Next, an ISS PCR could be performed on the yolk sac of those embryos to map the integration sites. We could create a database containing pictures of the lacZ expression with information on the trapped gene. In order to decrease the amount of animal housing, we could freeze the sperm of the founders. This sperm could then be used to resurrect the transgenic line. Finally, the long-held assumption that early embryogenesis is regulative has been tackled recently[5]. However, the definitive proof for a pre-patterning model will come from the identification of an uneven distribution of molecules within the zygote, reflecting the situation on non-mammals or from the differential expression of transcription factors within the early blastomeres driving differentiation towards one fate. Single cell transcriptome analysis could be used to discover a differential pattern of expression between early blastomeres. The probes should not only be enriched for genes expressed in early embryogenesis and stem cells such as the NIA 22K 60-mer oligo microarray but also not biased for the 3' region[128]. Namely, it has been shown that alternative splicing specifically in the proximal region can be implicated in the regulation of development[221]. It would be therefore interesting to incorporate splice variants within the gene microarrays and compare their relative contribution to early fate decision. Another interesting approach could be used to detect transiently active genes. As already discussed in the introduction, numerous genes show a transient activation and at specific embryonic stages[222, 223]. These transient wave-like activations are difficultly

Chapter 4. Development of a new lentiviral gene trap vector

analyzed by "snapshot" techniques such gene arrays[128]. Moreover, such studies are limited to the probes spotted on the microarray and do not probe genomic loci with yet unknown function. Thus, a more dynamic experimental setting is needed to follow the activation of transcriptional units during early embryogenesis. Lentiviral vector efficiently integrates into host genome within a few hours of infection. Moreover, integration is not random as it preferentially targets active transcriptional units[84]. Therefore, a new lentiviral gene trap vector could be developed. The short-lived nature of gene activation will impact on the choice of the reporter gene. It should be potent enough to be visualized rapidly and instable enough to wane rapidly. A destabilized version of eGFP, with a 2-hours half-life only, could be used[224]. To increase the strength of eGFP signal, we could clone a nuclear localization signal (nls) that will concentrate the molecules within the nucleus. This original gene trap construction can be microinjected into the perivitelline space of fertilized oocytes to produce founders carrying multiple trapped genes. Each integration site could then be precisely mapped using linear amplification PCR technique on tail DNA. These founders would produce F1 embryos that could be followed from the one-cell stage to the late blastocyst stage by time-lapse imaging and any expression of eGFP could be recorded. Every pattern of polarized eGFP expression could be easily linked to a trapped gene using integration site-specific PCR. However, is it reasonable to think that this approach could be used to track the emergence of gene activation during early development? According to a recent study, the number of newly activated genes that significantly increase between the one-cell stage and the two-cell stage is 3254, whereas this number drops to 1177 between the two-cell stage and the four-cell stage[128]. Providing that lentiviral-mediated transgenesis produces transgenic animals carrying on average 9 copies, we can calculate the amount of founders that we would need to trap those genes, considering also that only 20% of our vectors will efficiently trap genes. Thus, we will need around 1800 embryos to have a chance to trap once all the genes activated between the one-cell stage and the two-cell stage and 650 embryos for the second set of genes. These numbers are only rough estimations and probably underestimate the actual number of embryos needed. Obviously, these numbers are not compatible with in vivo settings. However, the blastomeres could show a differential display of gene activation, decreasing the number of activated gene per individual blastomere. Moreover, if a bias exists between early blastomeres, then their pattern of expression should diverge and encompasses many genes. Does an alternative experimental setting exist? A more reasonable approach could be to monitor in vitro the development of the injected embryos and to select the embryos presenting an eGFP polarization. Then, we could perform a LAM PCR on the blastocyst to retrieve the integration site. This will lead to candidate genes that could be further investigated. Alternatively, we could transfer only the blastocysts presenting a differential expression of eGFP and perform the experiments on F1 embryos, as discussed before. However, as we do not know the number of genes that could be differentially expressed between early blastomeres, if any, all the above-mentioned experimental designs could be used with their inherent advantages and pitfalls. For example, the use of F1 embryos is very interesting as all the integrant can be mapped in F0 and followed in F1 by PCR. Moreover, the germ-line transmission will be an attractive way to segregate the different proviruses to identify the one that give the phenotype. However, the number of mice can be insufficient to exclude that a differential display exists between early blastomeres.

Bibliography

1. Pfeifer A. Lentiviral transgenesis--a versatile tool for basic research and gene therapy. Curr Gene Ther 2006;6:535-42.
2. Palmiter RD, Brinster RL. Transgenic mice. Cell 1985;41:343-5.
3. Wall R. Transgenic livestock: progress and prospects for the future. Theriogenology 1996;45:57-68.
4. Hiiragi T, Alarcon VB, Fujimori T, et al. Where do we stand now? Mouse early embryo patterning meeting in Freiburg, Germany (2005). The International journal of developmental biology 2006;50:581-6; discussion 6-7.
5. Zernicka-Goetz M. The first cell-fate decisions in the mouse embryo: destiny is a matter of both chance and choice. Current opinion in genetics & development 2006;16:406-12.
6. Slack JMW. From Egg to Embryo: Determinative Events in Early Development. In: Cambridge University Press; 1983:1.
7. Alarcon VB, Marikawa Y. Unbiased contribution of the first two blastomeres to mouse blastocyst development. Molecular reproduction and development 2005;72:354-61.
8. Piotrowska K, Wianny F, Pedersen RA, Zernicka-Goetz M. Blastomeres arising from the first cleavage division have distinguishable fates in normal mouse development. Development (Cambridge, England) 2001;128:3739-48.
9. John M. Coffin SHH, Arnold E. Varmus. Retroviruses. In: Coffin JM, ed. Retroviruses. New York: Cold Spring Harbour Press; 1997:843.
10. Graham FL, van der Eb AJ. Transformation of rat cells by DNA of human adenovirus 5. Virology 1973;54:536-9.
11. Graham FL, van der Eb AJ. A new technique for the assay of infectivity of human adenovirus 5 DNA. Virology 1973;52:456-67.
12. Van der Eb AJ, Mulder C, Graham FL, Houweling A. Transformation with specific fragments of adenovirus DNAs. I. Isolation of specific fragments with transforming activity of adenovirus 2 and 5 DNA. Gene 1977;2:115-32.
13. Graham FL, Smiley J, Russell WC, Nairn R. Characteristics of a human cell line transformed by DNA from human adenovirus type 5. The Journal of general virology 1977;36:59-74.

14. Mak S, Mak I, Smiley JR, Graham FL. Tumorigenicity and viral gene expression in rat cells transformed by Ad 12 virions or by the EcoRI c fragment of Ad 12 DNA. Virology 1979;98:456-60.
15. van der Eb AJ, Graham FL. Assay of transforming activity of tumor virus DNA. Methods in enzymology 1980;65:826-39.
16. Bacchetti S, Graham FL. Transfer of the gene for thymidine kinase to thymidine kinase-deficient human cells by purified herpes simplex viral DNA. Proc Natl Acad Sci U S A 1977;74:1590-4.
17. Bacchetti S, Graham FL. DNA-mediated transfer of herpes simplex virus TK gene to human TK- cells: properties of the transformed lines. IARC scientific publications 1978:495-9.
18. Goff SP, Berg P. Construction of hybrid viruses containing SV40 and lambda phage DNA segments and their propagation in cultured monkey cells. Cell 1976;9:695-705.
19. Lim B, Williams DA, Orkin SH. Retrovirus-mediated gene transfer of human adenosine deaminase: expression of functional enzyme in murine hematopoietic stem cells in vivo. Molecular and cellular biology 1987;7:3459-65.
20. Keller G, Paige C, Gilboa E, Wagner EF. Expression of a foreign gene in myeloid and lymphoid cells derived from multipotent haematopoietic precursors. Nature 1985;318:149-54.
21. van der Putten H, Botteri FM, Miller AD, et al. Efficient insertion of genes into the mouse germ line via retroviral vectors. Proc Natl Acad Sci U S A 1985;82:6148-52.
22. Miller AD, Ong ES, Rosenfeld MG, Verma IM, Evans RM. Infectious and selectable retrovirus containing an inducible rat growth hormone minigene. Science 1984;225:993-8.
23. Roe T, Reynolds TC, Yu G, Brown PO. Integration of murine leukemia virus DNA depends on mitosis. The EMBO journal 1993;12:2099-108.
24. Lewis PF, Emerman M. Passage through mitosis is required for oncoretroviruses but not for the human immunodeficiency virus. J Virol 1994;68:510-6.
25. Lewis P, Hensel M, Emerman M. Human immunodeficiency virus infection of cells arrested in the cell cycle. The EMBO journal 1992;11:3053-8.

26. Naldini L, Blomer U, Gallay P, et al. In vivo gene delivery and stable transduction of nondividing cells by a lentiviral vector. Science 1996;272:263-7.
27. Gallay P, Stitt V, Mundy C, Oettinger M, Trono D. Role of the karyopherin pathway in human immunodeficiency virus type 1 nuclear import. J Virol 1996;70:1027-32.
28. Bukrinsky MI, Sharova N, Dempsey MP, et al. Active nuclear import of human immunodeficiency virus type 1 preintegration complexes. Proc Natl Acad Sci U S A 1992;89:6580-4.
29. Bukrinsky MI, Haggerty S, Dempsey MP, et al. A nuclear localization signal within HIV-1 matrix protein that governs infection of nondividing cells. Nature 1993;365:666-9.
30. Gallay P, Hope T, Chin D, Trono D. HIV-1 infection of nondividing cells through the recognition of integrase by the importin/karyopherin pathway. Proc Natl Acad Sci U S A 1997;94:9825-30.
31. Heinzinger NK, Bukrinsky MI, Haggerty SA, et al. The Vpr protein of human immunodeficiency virus type 1 influences nuclear localization of viral nucleic acids in nondividing host cells. Proc Natl Acad Sci U S A 1994;91:7311-5.
32. von Schwedler U, Kornbluth RS, Trono D. The nuclear localization signal of the matrix protein of human immunodeficiency virus type 1 allows the establishment of infection in macrophages and quiescent T lymphocytes. Proc Natl Acad Sci U S A 1994;91:6992-6.
33. Burns JC, Friedmann T, Driever W, Burrascano M, Yee JK. Vesicular stomatitis virus G glycoprotein pseudotyped retroviral vectors: concentration to very high titer and efficient gene transfer into mammalian and nonmammalian cells. Proc Natl Acad Sci U S A 1993;90:8033-7.
34. Reiser J, Harmison G, Kluepfel-Stahl S, Brady RO, Karlsson S, Schubert M. Transduction of nondividing cells using pseudotyped defective high-titer HIV type 1 particles. Proc Natl Acad Sci U S A 1996;93:15266-71.
35. Zufferey R, Nagy D, Mandel RJ, Naldini L, Trono D. Multiply attenuated lentiviral vector achieves efficient gene delivery in vivo. Nature biotechnology 1997;15:871-5.
36. Bieniasz PD, Grdina TA, Bogerd HP, Cullen BR. Highly divergent lentiviral Tat proteins activate viral gene expression by a common mechanism. Molecular and cellular biology 1999;19:4592-9.

37. Miyoshi H, Blomer U, Takahashi M, Gage FH, Verma IM. Development of a self-inactivating lentivirus vector. J Virol 1998;72:8150-7.
38. Zufferey R, Dull T, Mandel RJ, et al. Self-inactivating lentivirus vector for safe and efficient in vivo gene delivery. J Virol 1998;72:9873-80.
39. Dull T, Zufferey R, Kelly M, et al. A third-generation lentivirus vector with a conditional packaging system. J Virol 1998;72:8463-71.
40. Trono D. Lentiviral vectors: turning a deadly foe into a therapeutic agent. Gene therapy 2000;7:20-3.
41. Geyer PK, Spana C, Corces VG. On the molecular mechanism of gypsy-induced mutations at the yellow locus of Drosophila melanogaster. The EMBO journal 1986;5:2657-62.
42. Gerasimova TI, Byrd K, Corces VG. A chromatin insulator determines the nuclear localization of DNA. Molecular cell 2000;6:1025-35.
43. Chung JH, Whiteley M, Felsenfeld G. A 5' element of the chicken beta-globin domain serves as an insulator in human erythroid cells and protects against position effect in Drosophila. Cell 1993;74:505-14.
44. Pikaart MJ, Recillas-Targa F, Felsenfeld G. Loss of transcriptional activity of a transgene is accompanied by DNA methylation and histone deacetylation and is prevented by insulators. Genes & development 1998;12:2852-62.
45. Baniahmad A, Steiner C, Kohne AC, Renkawitz R. Modular structure of a chicken lysozyme silencer: involvement of an unusual thyroid hormone receptor binding site. Cell 1990;61:505-14.
46. Chung JH, Bell AC, Felsenfeld G. Characterization of the chicken beta-globin insulator. Proc Natl Acad Sci U S A 1997;94:575-80.
47. Bell AC, West AG, Felsenfeld G. The protein CTCF is required for the enhancer blocking activity of vertebrate insulators. Cell 1999;98:387-96.
48. Bell AC, Felsenfeld G. Methylation of a CTCF-dependent boundary controls imprinted expression of the Igf2 gene. Nature 2000;405:482-5.
49. Hark AT, Schoenherr CJ, Katz DJ, Ingram RS, Levorse JM, Tilghman SM. CTCF mediates methylation-sensitive enhancer-blocking activity at the H19/Igf2 locus. Nature 2000;405:486-9.
50. Yusufzai TM, Tagami H, Nakatani Y, Felsenfeld G. CTCF tethers an insulator to subnuclear sites, suggesting shared insulator mechanisms across species. Molecular cell 2004;13:291-8.

51. Brown SA, Fleury-Olela F, Nagoshi E, et al. The period length of fibroblast circadian gene expression varies widely among human individuals. PLoS Biol 2005;3:e338.
52. Lopes L, Dewannieux M, Gileadi U, et al. Immunization with a lentivector that targets tumor antigen expression to dendritic cells induces potent CD8+ and CD4+ T-cell responses. J Virol 2008;82:86-95.
53. Han XD, Lin C, Chang J, Sadelain M, Kan YW. Fetal gene therapy of alpha-thalassemia in a mouse model. Proc Natl Acad Sci U S A 2007;104:9007-11.
54. Logg CR, Logg A, Matusik RJ, Bochner BH, Kasahara N. Tissue-specific transcriptional targeting of a replication-competent retroviral vector. J Virol 2002;76:12783-91.
55. Gossen M, Bujard H. Tight control of gene expression in mammalian cells by tetracycline-responsive promoters. Proc Natl Acad Sci U S A 1992;89:5547-51.
56. Haack K, Cockrell AS, Ma H, et al. Transactivator and structurally optimized inducible lentiviral vectors. Mol Ther 2004;10:585-96.
57. Gossen M, Freundlieb S, Bender G, Muller G, Hillen W, Bujard H. Transcriptional activation by tetracyclines in mammalian cells. Science 1995;268:1766-9.
58. Regulier E, Pereira de Almeida L, Sommer B, Aebischer P, Deglon N. Dose-dependent neuroprotective effect of ciliary neurotrophic factor delivered via tetracycline-regulated lentiviral vectors in the quinolinic acid rat model of Huntington's disease. Human gene therapy 2002;13:1981-90.
59. Barde I, Zanta-Boussif MA, Paisant S, et al. Efficient control of gene expression in the hematopoietic system using a single Tet-on inducible lentiviral vector. Mol Ther 2006;13:382-90.
60. Vigna E, Amendola M, Benedicenti F, Simmons AD, Follenzi A, Naldini L. Efficient Tet-dependent expression of human factor IX in vivo by a new self-regulating lentiviral vector. Mol Ther 2005;11:763-75.
61. Fire A, Xu S, Montgomery MK, Kostas SA, Driver SE, Mello CC. Potent and specific genetic interference by double-stranded RNA in Caenorhabditis elegans. Nature 1998;391:806-11.
62. Elbashir SM, Harborth J, Lendeckel W, Yalcin A, Weber K, Tuschl T. Duplexes of 21-nucleotide RNAs mediate RNA interference in cultured mammalian cells. Nature 2001;411:494-8.

63.   Kennerdell JR, Carthew RW. Heritable gene silencing in Drosophila using double-stranded RNA. Nature biotechnology 2000;18:896-8.
64.   Miyagishi M, Taira K. U6 promoter-driven siRNAs with four uridine 3' overhangs efficiently suppress targeted gene expression in mammalian cells. Nature biotechnology 2002;20:497-500.
65.   Brummelkamp TR, Bernards R, Agami R. A system for stable expression of short interfering RNAs in mammalian cells. Science 2002;296:550-3.
66.   Meister G, Tuschl T. Mechanisms of gene silencing by double-stranded RNA. Nature 2004;431:343-9.
67.   Meister G. Molecular biology. RNA interference in the nucleus. Science 2008;321:496-7.
68.   Wiznerowicz M, Szulc J, Trono D. Tuning silence: conditional systems for RNA interference. Nat Methods 2006;3:682-8.
69.   Sandy P, Ventura A, Jacks T. Mammalian RNAi: a practical guide. Biotechniques 2005;39:215-24.
70.   Wiznerowicz M, Trono D. Conditional suppression of cellular genes: lentivirus vector-mediated drug-inducible RNA interference. J Virol 2003;77:8957-61.
71.   Szulc J, Wiznerowicz M, Sauvain MO, Trono D, Aebischer P. A versatile tool for conditional gene expression and knockdown. Nat Methods 2006;3:109-16.
72.   Filipowicz W, Bhattacharyya SN, Sonenberg N. Mechanisms of post-transcriptional regulation by microRNAs: are the answers in sight? Nature reviews 2008;9:102-14.
73.   Shin KJ, Wall EA, Zavzavadjian JR, et al. A single lentiviral vector platform for microRNA-based conditional RNA interference and coordinated transgene expression. Proc Natl Acad Sci U S A 2006;103:13759-64.
74.   Copreni E, Penzo M, Carrabino S, Conese M. Lentivirus-mediated gene transfer to the respiratory epithelium: a promising approach to gene therapy of cystic fibrosis. Gene therapy 2004;11 Suppl 1:S67-75.
75.   Nguyen TH, Aubert D, Bellodi-Privato M, et al. Critical assessment of lifelong phenotype correction in hyperbilirubinemic Gunn rats after retroviral mediated gene transfer. Gene therapy 2007;14:1270-7.
76.   Nguyen TH, Birraux J, Wildhaber B, et al. Ex vivo lentivirus transduction and immediate transplantation of uncultured hepatocytes for treating hyperbilirubinemic Gunn rat. Transplantation 2006;82:794-803.

77. Kafri T, Blomer U, Peterson DA, Gage FH, Verma IM. Sustained expression of genes delivered directly into liver and muscle by lentiviral vectors. Nat Genet 1997;17:314-7.
78. Cavazzana-Calvo M, Hacein-Bey S, de Saint Basile G, et al. Gene therapy of human severe combined immunodeficiency (SCID)-X1 disease. Science 2000;288:669-72.
79. Hacein-Bey-Abina S, Von Kalle C, Schmidt M, et al. LMO2-associated clonal T cell proliferation in two patients after gene therapy for SCID-X1. Science 2003;302:415-9.
80. Hacein-Bey-Abina S, Garrigue A, Wang GP, et al. Insertional oncogenesis in 4 patients after retrovirus-mediated gene therapy of SCID-X1. The Journal of clinical investigation 2008.
81. Howe SJ, Mansour MR, Schwarzwaelder K, et al. Insertional mutagenesis combined with acquired somatic mutations causes leukemogenesis following gene therapy of SCID-X1 patients. The Journal of clinical investigation 2008.
82. Pike-Overzet K, van der Burg M, Wagemaker G, van Dongen JJ, Staal FJ. New insights and unresolved issues regarding insertional mutagenesis in X-linked SCID gene therapy. Mol Ther 2007;15:1910-6.
83. Bushman FD. Retroviral integration and human gene therapy. The Journal of clinical investigation 2007;117:2083-6.
84. Mitchell RS, Beitzel BF, Schroder AR, et al. Retroviral DNA integration: ASLV, HIV, and MLV show distinct target site preferences. PLoS Biol 2004;2:E234.
85. Lewinski MK, Yamashita M, Emerman M, et al. Retroviral DNA integration: viral and cellular determinants of target-site selection. PLoS pathogens 2006;2:e60.
86. Marshall HM, Ronen K, Berry C, et al. Role of PSIP1/LEDGF/p75 in lentiviral infectivity and integration targeting. PLoS ONE 2007;2:e1340.
87. Wang GP, Ciuffi A, Leipzig J, Berry CC, Bushman FD. HIV integration site selection: analysis by massively parallel pyrosequencing reveals association with epigenetic modifications. Genome Res 2007;17:1186-94.
88. Park F. Lentiviral vectors: are they the future of animal transgenesis? Physiological genomics 2007;31:159-73.
89. Gordon K, Ruddle FH. Gene transfer into mouse embryos. Dev Biol (N Y 1985) 1986;4:1-36.

90. Jaenisch R, Mintz B. Simian virus 40 DNA sequences in DNA of healthy adult mice derived from preimplantation blastocysts injected with viral DNA. Proc Natl Acad Sci U S A 1974;71:1250-4.
91. Stuhlmann H, Jaenisch R, Mulligan RC. Transfer of a mutant dihydrofolate reductase gene into pre- and postimplantation mouse embryos by a replication-competent retrovirus vector. J Virol 1989;63:4857-65.
92. Jaenisch R, Fan H, Croker B. Infection of preimplantation mouse embryos and of newborn mice with leukemia virus: tissue distribution of viral DNA and RNA and leukemogenesis in the adult animal. Proc Natl Acad Sci U S A 1975;72:4008-12.
93. Miller AR, Skotzko MJ, Rhoades K, et al. Simultaneous use of two retroviral vectors in human gene marking trials: feasibility and potential applications. Human gene therapy 1992;3:619-24.
94. Foresman MD, Nelson DM, McIvor RS. Correction of purine nucleoside phosphorylase deficiency by retroviral-mediated gene transfer in mouse S49 T cell lymphoma: a model for gene therapy of T cell immunodeficiency. Human gene therapy 1992;3:625-31.
95. Jahner D, Jaenisch R. Retrovirus-induced de novo methylation of flanking host sequences correlates with gene inactivity. Nature 1985;315:594-7.
96. Brinster RL. The effect of cells transferred into the mouse blastocyst on subsequent development. The Journal of experimental medicine 1974;140:1049-56.
97. Gordon JW, Scangos GA, Plotkin DJ, Barbosa JA, Ruddle FH. Genetic transformation of mouse embryos by microinjection of purified DNA. Proc Natl Acad Sci U S A 1980;77:7380-4.
98. Brinster RL, Chen HY, Trumbauer M, Senear AW, Warren R, Palmiter RD. Somatic expression of herpes thymidine kinase in mice following injection of a fusion gene into eggs. Cell 1981;27:223-31.
99. Wall RJ. Pronuclear microinjection. Cloning and stem cells 2001;3:209-20.
100. Moffat AS. Improving gene transfer into livestock. Science 1998;282:1619-20.
101. Lois C, Hong EJ, Pease S, Brown EJ, Baltimore D. Germline transmission and tissue-specific expression of transgenes delivered by lentiviral vectors. Science 2002;295:868-72.

102. Okada Y, Ueshin Y, Isotani A, et al. Complementation of placental defects and embryonic lethality by trophoblast-specific lentiviral gene transfer. Nature biotechnology 2007;25:233-7.
103. Hofmann A, Kessler B, Ewerling S, et al. Efficient transgenesis in farm animals by lentiviral vectors. EMBO Rep 2003;4:1054-60.
104. Gao X, Zhang P. Transgenic RNA interference in mice. Physiology (Bethesda, Md 2007;22:161-6.
105. Tiscornia G, Singer O, Ikawa M, Verma IM. A general method for gene knockdown in mice by using lentiviral vectors expressing small interfering RNA. Proc Natl Acad Sci U S A 2003;100:1844-8.
106. Rubinson DA, Dillon CP, Kwiatkowski AV, et al. A lentivirus-based system to functionally silence genes in primary mammalian cells, stem cells and transgenic mice by RNA interference. Nat Genet 2003;33:401-6.
107. Kissler S, Stern P, Takahashi K, Hunter K, Peterson LB, Wicker LS. In vivo RNA interference demonstrates a role for Nramp1 in modifying susceptibility to type 1 diabetes. Nat Genet 2006;38:479-83.
108. Tiscornia G, Tergaonkar V, Galimi F, Verma IM. CRE recombinase-inducible RNA interference mediated by lentiviral vectors. Proc Natl Acad Sci U S A 2004;101:7347-51.
109. Feil R, Wagner J, Metzger D, Chambon P. Regulation of Cre recombinase activity by mutated estrogen receptor ligand-binding domains. Biochemical and biophysical research communications 1997;237:752-7.
110. Rossant J. Stem cells and lineage development in the mammalian blastocyst. Reproduction, fertility, and development 2007;19:111-8.
111. Nagy A, Gocza E, Diaz EM, et al. Embryonic stem cells alone are able to support fetal development in the mouse. Development (Cambridge, England) 1990;110:815-21.
112. Li X, Yu Y, Wei W, et al. Simple and efficient production of mice derived from embryonic stem cells aggregated with tetraploid embryos. Molecular reproduction and development 2005;71:154-8.
113. Eggan K, Akutsu H, Loring J, et al. Hybrid vigor, fetal overgrowth, and viability of mice derived by nuclear cloning and tetraploid embryo complementation. Proc Natl Acad Sci U S A 2001;98:6209-14.
114. Ventura A, Meissner A, Dillon CP, et al. Cre-lox-regulated conditional RNA interference from transgenes. Proc Natl Acad Sci U S A 2004;101:10380-5.

115. Gotta M, Ahringer J. Axis determination in C. elegans: initiating and transducing polarity. Current opinion in genetics & development 2001;11:367-73.
116. King ML, Zhou Y, Bubunenko M. Polarizing genetic information in the egg: RNA localization in the frog oocyte. Bioessays 1999;21:546-57.
117. Rossant J, Tam PP. Emerging asymmetry and embryonic patterning in early mouse development. Dev Cell 2004;7:155-64.
118. Huynh JR, St Johnston D. The origin of asymmetry: early polarisation of the Drosophila germline cyst and oocyte. Curr Biol 2004;14:R438-49.
119. St Johnston D, Nusslein-Volhard C. The origin of pattern and polarity in the Drosophila embryo. Cell 1992;68:201-19.
120. Ephrussi A, St Johnston D. Seeing is believing: the bicoid morphogen gradient matures. Cell 2004;116:143-52.
121. Zernicka-Goetz M. Cleavage pattern and emerging asymmetry of the mouse embryo. Nat Rev Mol Cell Biol 2005;6:919-28.
122. Tarkowski AK. Experiments on the development of isolated blastomers of mouse eggs. Nature 1959;184:1286-7.
123. Tsunoda Y, McLaren A. Effect of various procedures on the viability of mouse embryos containing half the normal number of blastomeres. Journal of reproduction and fertility 1983;69:315-22.
124. Tarkowski AK, Wroblewska J. Development of blastomeres of mouse eggs isolated at the 4- and 8-cell stage. Journal of embryology and experimental morphology 1967;18:155-80.
125. Piotrowska-Nitsche K, Zernicka-Goetz M. Spatial arrangement of individual 4-cell stage blastomeres and the order in which they are generated correlate with blastocyst pattern in the mouse embryo. Mechanisms of development 2005;122:487-500.
126. Piotrowska-Nitsche K, Perea-Gomez A, Haraguchi S, Zernicka-Goetz M. Four-cell stage mouse blastomeres have different developmental properties. Development (Cambridge, England) 2005;132:479-90.
127. Plusa B, Hadjantonakis AK, Gray D, et al. The first cleavage of the mouse zygote predicts the blastocyst axis. Nature 2005;434:391-5.
128. Hamatani T, Ko M, Yamada M, et al. Global gene expression profiling of preimplantation embryos. Hum Cell 2006;19:98-117.
129. Bachvarova R, De Leon V, Johnson A, Kaplan G, Paynton BV. Changes in total RNA, polyadenylated RNA, and actin mRNA during meiotic maturation of mouse oocytes. Developmental biology 1985;108:325-31.

130. Piko L, Clegg KB. Quantitative changes in total RNA, total poly(A), and ribosomes in early mouse embryos. Developmental biology 1982;89:362-78.
131. Schultz RM. The molecular foundations of the maternal to zygotic transition in the preimplantation embryo. Human reproduction update 2002;8:323-31.
132. Aoki F, Worrad DM, Schultz RM. Regulation of transcriptional activity during the first and second cell cycles in the preimplantation mouse embryo. Developmental biology 1997;181:296-307.
133. Latham KE, Garrels JI, Chang C, Solter D. Quantitative analysis of protein synthesis in mouse embryos. I. Extensive reprogramming at the one- and two-cell stages. Development (Cambridge, England) 1991;112:921-32.
134. Nothias JY, Majumder S, Kaneko KJ, DePamphilis ML. Regulation of gene expression at the beginning of mammalian development. The Journal of biological chemistry 1995;270:22077-80.
135. Thompson EM, Legouy E, Renard JP. Mouse embryos do not wait for the MBT: chromatin and RNA polymerase remodeling in genome activation at the onset of development. Developmental genetics 1998;22:31-42.
136. Russell WL, Russell LB, Kelly EM. Radiation dose rate and mutation frequency. Science 1958;128:1546-50.
137. Bode VC, McDonald JD, Guenet JL, Simon D. hph-1: a mouse mutant with hereditary hyperphenylalaninemia induced by ethylnitrosourea mutagenesis. Genetics 1988;118:299-305.
138. Russell WL, Kelly EM, Hunsicker PR, Bangham JW, Maddux SC, Phipps EL. Specific-locus test shows ethylnitrosourea to be the most potent mutagen in the mouse. Proc Natl Acad Sci U S A 1979;76:5818-9.
139. McDonald JD, Beier D. ENU mutagenesis in the mouse. Current protocols in human genetics / editorial board, Jonathan L Haines [et al 2004;Chapter 15:Unit 15 4.
140. Anderson KV. Finding the genes that direct mammalian development : ENU mutagenesis in the mouse. Trends Genet 2000;16:99-102.
141. Vitaterna MH, King DP, Chang AM, et al. Mutagenesis and mapping of a mouse gene, Clock, essential for circadian behavior. Science 1994;264:719-25.
142. Soriano P. Gene targeting in ES cells. Annual review of neuroscience 1995;18:1-18.

143. Capecchi MR. Gene targeting in mice: functional analysis of the mammalian genome for the twenty-first century. Nature reviews 2005;6:507-12.
144. Stanford WL, Cohn JB, Cordes SP. Gene-trap mutagenesis: past, present and beyond. Nature reviews 2001;2:756-68.
145. Kuehn MR, Bradley A, Robertson EJ, Evans MJ. A potential animal model for Lesch-Nyhan syndrome through introduction of HPRT mutations into mice. Nature 1987;326:295-8.
146. Hooper M, Hardy K, Handyside A, Hunter S, Monk M. HPRT-deficient (Lesch-Nyhan) mouse embryos derived from germline colonization by cultured cells. Nature 1987;326:292-5.
147. Bradley A, Evans M, Kaufman MH, Robertson E. Formation of germ-line chimaeras from embryo-derived teratocarcinoma cell lines. Nature 1984;309:255-6.
148. Gossler A, Joyner AL, Rossant J, Skarnes WC. Mouse embryonic stem cells and reporter constructs to detect developmentally regulated genes. Science 1989;244:463-5.
149. Friedrich G, Soriano P. Promoter traps in embryonic stem cells: a genetic screen to identify and mutate developmental genes in mice. Genes & development 1991;5:1513-23.
150. von Melchner H, DeGregori JV, Rayburn H, Reddy S, Friedel C, Ruley HE. Selective disruption of genes expressed in totipotent embryonal stem cells. Genes & development 1992;6:919-27.
151. Hansen J, Floss T, Van Sloun P, et al. A large-scale, gene-driven mutagenesis approach for the functional analysis of the mouse genome. Proc Natl Acad Sci U S A 2003;100:9918-22.
152. Pfeifer A. Lentiviral transgenesis. Transgenic research 2004;13:513-22.
153. Schmidt M, Zickler P, Hoffmann G, et al. Polyclonal long-term repopulating stem cell clones in a primate model. Blood 2002;100:2737-43.
154. Ewing B, Hillier L, Wendl MC, Green P. Base-calling of automated sequencer traces using phred. I. Accuracy assessment. Genome Res 1998;8:175-85.
155. Kent WJ. BLAT--the BLAST-like alignment tool. Genome Res 2002;12:656-64.
156. Zhang Z, Schwartz S, Wagner L, Miller W. A greedy algorithm for aligning DNA sequences. J Comput Biol 2000;7:203-14.

157. Ying QL, Nichols J, Evans EP, Smith AG. Changing potency by spontaneous fusion. Nature 2002;416:545-8.
158. Vandesompele J, De Preter K, Pattyn F, et al. Accurate normalization of real-time quantitative RT-PCR data by geometric averaging of multiple internal control genes. Genome Biol 2002;3:RESEARCH0034.
159. Oka M, Chang LJ, Costantini F, Terada N. Lentiviral vector-mediated gene transfer in embryonic stem cells. Methods in molecular biology (Clifton, NJ 2006;329:273-81.
160. Stuhlmann H, Jahner D, Jaenisch R. Infectivity and methylation of retroviral genomes is correlated with expression in the animal. Cell 1981;26:221-32.
161. Wolf D, Goff SP. TRIM28 mediates primer binding site-targeted silencing of murine leukemia virus in embryonic cells. Cell 2007;131:46-57.
162. Vandegraaff N, Kumar R, Burrell CJ, Li P. Kinetics of human immunodeficiency virus type 1 (HIV) DNA integration in acutely infected cells as determined using a novel assay for detection of integrated HIV DNA. J Virol 2001;75:11253-60.
163. Nagy A, Vintersten K. Murine embryonic stem cells. Methods in enzymology 2006;418:3-21.
164. Molyneaux K, Wylie C. Primordial germ cell migration. The International journal of developmental biology 2004;48:537-44.
165. Donovan PJ. The germ cell--the mother of all stem cells. The International journal of developmental biology 1998;42:1043-50.
166. Starz-Gaiano M, Cho NK, Forbes A, Lehmann R. Spatially restricted activity of a Drosophila lipid phosphatase guides migrating germ cells. Development (Cambridge, England) 2001;128:983-91.
167. Raz E. Primordial germ-cell development: the zebrafish perspective. Nature reviews 2003;4:690-700.
168. Pfingsten JS, Costantino DA, Kieft JS. Structural basis for ribosome recruitment and manipulation by a viral IRES RNA. Science 2006;314:1450-4.
169. Weber EL, Cannon PM. Promoter choice for retroviral vectors: transcriptional strength versus trans-activation potential. Human gene therapy 2007;18:849-60.
170. Goff SP. Retrovirus restriction factors. Molecular cell 2004;16:849-59.

171. Nisole S, Stoye JP, Saib A. TRIM family proteins: retroviral restriction and antiviral defence. Nat Rev Microbiol 2005;3:799-808.
172. Rhodes DA, de Bono B, Trowsdale J. Relationship between SPRY and B30.2 protein domains. Evolution of a component of immune defence? Immunology 2005;116:411-7.
173. Bieniasz PD. Intrinsic immunity: a front-line defense against viral attack. Nature immunology 2004;5:1109-15.
174. Si Z, Vandegraaff N, O'Huigin C, et al. Evolution of a cytoplasmic tripartite motif (TRIM) protein in cows that restricts retroviral infection. Proc Natl Acad Sci U S A 2006;103:7454-9.
175. Conner SJ, Lefievre L, Hughes DC, Barratt CL. Cracking the egg: increased complexity in the zona pellucida. Human reproduction (Oxford, England) 2005;20:1148-52.
176. Hacein-Bey-Abina S, von Kalle C, Schmidt M, et al. A serious adverse event after successful gene therapy for X-linked severe combined immunodeficiency. N Engl J Med 2003;348:255-6.
177. Noguchi M, Yi H, Rosenblatt HM, et al. Interleukin-2 receptor gamma chain mutation results in X-linked severe combined immunodeficiency in humans. Cell 1993;73:147-57.
178. Sugamura K, Asao H, Kondo M, et al. The interleukin-2 receptor gamma chain: its role in the multiple cytokine receptor complexes and T cell development in XSCID. Annual review of immunology 1996;14:179-205.
179. Buckley RH, Schiff SE, Schiff RI, et al. Hematopoietic stem-cell transplantation for the treatment of severe combined immunodeficiency. N Engl J Med 1999;340:508-16.
180. Bushman FD. Integration site selection by lentiviruses: biology and possible control. Current topics in microbiology and immunology 2002;261:165-77.
181. Bauer G, Dao MA, Case SS, et al. In vivo biosafety model to assess the risk of adverse events from retroviral and lentiviral vectors. Mol Ther 2008;16:1308-15.
182. Peaston AE, Evsikov AV, Graber JH, et al. Retrotransposons regulate host genes in mouse oocytes and preimplantation embryos. Dev Cell 2004;7:597-606.
183. Waterston RH, Lindblad-Toh K, Birney E, et al. Initial sequencing and comparative analysis of the mouse genome. Nature 2002;420:520-62.

184. Mattick JS. A new paradigm for developmental biology. The Journal of experimental biology 2007;210:1526-47.
185. Kazazian HH, Jr. Mobile elements: drivers of genome evolution. Science 2004;303:1626-32.
186. Santos F, Hendrich B, Reik W, Dean W. Dynamic reprogramming of DNA methylation in the early mouse embryo. Developmental biology 2002;241:172-82.
187. Bestor TH. Cytosine methylation mediates sexual conflict. Trends Genet 2003;19:185-90.
188. Li E. Chromatin modification and epigenetic reprogramming in mammalian development. Nature reviews 2002;3:662-73.
189. Bushman F, Lewinski M, Ciuffi A, et al. Genome-wide analysis of retroviral DNA integration. Nat Rev Microbiol 2005;3:848-58.
190. Taddei A, Hediger F, Neumann FR, Gasser SM. The function of nuclear architecture: a genetic approach. Annual review of genetics 2004;38:305-45.
191. Gasser SM. Positions of potential: nuclear organization and gene expression. Cell 2001;104:639-42.
192. Cremer T, Cremer C. Chromosome territories, nuclear architecture and gene regulation in mammalian cells. Nature reviews 2001;2:292-301.
193. Casolari JM, Brown CR, Komili S, West J, Hieronymus H, Silver PA. Genome-wide localization of the nuclear transport machinery couples transcriptional status and nuclear organization. Cell 2004;117:427-39.
194. Komili S, Silver PA. Coupling and coordination in gene expression processes: a systems biology view. Nature reviews 2008;9:38-48.
195. Akhtar A, Gasser SM. The nuclear envelope and transcriptional control. Nature reviews 2007;8:507-17.
196. Schneider R, Grosschedl R. Dynamics and interplay of nuclear architecture, genome organization, and gene expression. Genes & development 2007;21:3027-43.
197. Heintz N. BAC to the future: the use of bac transgenic mice for neuroscience research. Nat Rev Neurosci 2001;2:861-70.
198. Vogel G. Embryology. Embryologists polarized over early cell fate determination. Science 2005;308:782-3.
199. Chroscicka A, Komorowski S, Maleszewski M. Both blastomeres of the mouse 2-cell embryo contribute to the embryonic portion of the blastocyst. Molecular reproduction and development 2004;68:308-12.

200. Motosugi N, Bauer T, Polanski Z, Solter D, Hiiragi T. Polarity of the mouse embryo is established at blastocyst and is not prepatterned. Genes & development 2005;19:1081-92.
201. Fujimori T, Kurotaki Y, Miyazaki J, Nabeshima Y. Analysis of cell lineage in two- and four-cell mouse embryos. Development (Cambridge, England) 2003;130:5113-22.
202. Kurotaki Y, Hatta K, Nakao K, Nabeshima Y, Fujimori T. Blastocyst axis is specified independently of early cell lineage but aligns with the ZP shape. Science 2007;316:719-23.
203. Sauvain MO, Dorr AP, Stevenson B, et al. Genotypic features of lentivirus transgenic mice. J Virol 2008;82:7111-9.
204. Tam PP, Loebel DA. Gene function in mouse embryogenesis: get set for gastrulation. Nature reviews 2007;8:368-81.
205. Schatten G, Donovan P. Embryology: plane talk. Nature 2004;430:301-2.
206. Rossant J, Tam PPL. Emerging asymmetry and embryonic patterning in early mouse development. Developmental cell 2004;7:155-64.
207. Torres-Padilla ME, Parfitt DE, Kouzarides T, Zernicka-Goetz M. Histone arginine methylation regulates pluripotency in the early mouse embryo. Nature 2007;445:214-8.
208. Mitsui K, Tokuzawa Y, Itoh H, et al. The homeoprotein Nanog is required for maintenance of pluripotency in mouse epiblast and ES cells. Cell 2003;113:631-42.
209. Avilion AA, Nicolis SK, Pevny LH, Perez L, Vivian N, Lovell-Badge R. Multipotent cell lineages in early mouse development depend on SOX2 function. Genes & development 2003;17:126-40.
210. Rasmussen TP. Developmentally-poised chromatin of embryonic stem cells. Front Biosci 2008;13:1568-77.
211. Bernstein E, Kim SY, Carmell MA, et al. Dicer is essential for mouse development. Nat Genet 2003;35:215-7.
212. Pace AJ, Lee E, Athirakul K, Coffman TM, O'Brien DA, Koller BH. Failure of spermatogenesis in mouse lines deficient in the Na(+)-K(+)-2Cl(-) cotransporter. The Journal of clinical investigation 2000;105:441-50.
213. Macara IG. Parsing the polarity code. Nat Rev Mol Cell Biol 2004;5:220-31.

214. Plusa B, Frankenberg S, Chalmers A, et al. Downregulation of Par3 and aPKC function directs cells towards the ICM in the preimplantation mouse embryo. Journal of cell science 2005;118:505-15.
215. De Palma M, Montini E, de Sio FRS, et al. Promoter trapping reveals significant differences in integration site selection between MLV and HIV vectors in primary hematopoietic cells. Blood 2005;105:2307-15.
216. Martinez-Salas E. Internal ribosome entry site biology and its use in expression vectors. Current opinion in biotechnology 1999;10:458-64.
217. Mallo M. Controlled gene activation and inactivation in the mouse. Front Biosci 2006;11:313-27.
218. Wiles MV, Vauti F, Otte J, et al. Establishment of a gene-trap sequence tag library to generate mutant mice from embryonic stem cells. Nat Genet 2000;24:13-4.
219. To C, Epp T, Reid T, et al. The Centre for Modeling Human Disease Gene Trap resource. Nucleic acids research 2004;32:D557-9.
220. Skarnes WC, von Melchner H, Wurst W, et al. A public gene trap resource for mouse functional genomics. Nat Genet 2004;36:543-4.
221. Yeo GW, Van Nostrand E, Holste D, Poggio T, Burge CB. Identification and analysis of alternative splicing events conserved in human and mouse. Proc Natl Acad Sci U S A 2005;102:2850-5.
222. Schier AF. The maternal-zygotic transition: death and birth of RNAs. Science 2007;316:406-7.
223. Zeng F, Baldwin DA, Schultz RM. Transcript profiling during preimplantation mouse development. Developmental biology 2004;272:483-96.
224. Li X, Zhao X, Fang Y, et al. Generation of destabilized green fluorescent protein as a transcription reporter. The Journal of biological chemistry 1998;273:34970-5.

Addendum

Lentiviral mediated transgenesis

MODUS OPERANDI

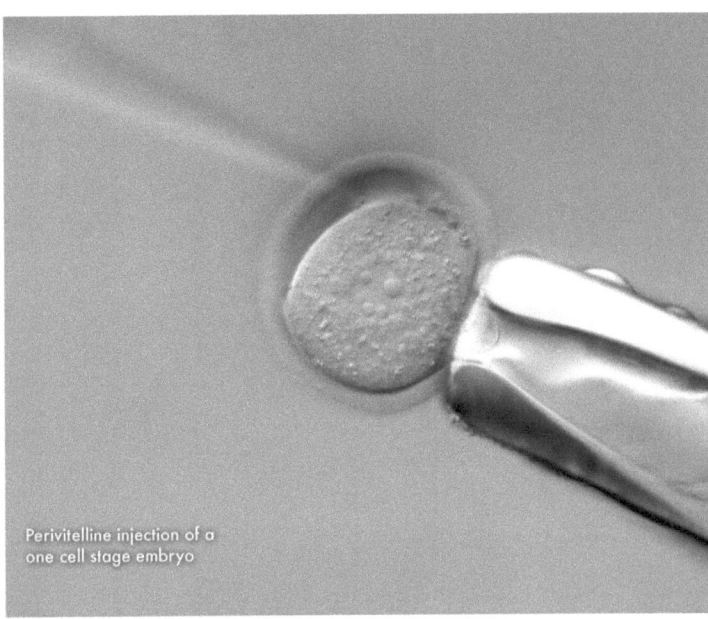

Perivitelline injection of a one cell stage embryo

Perivitelline injection

Introduction

Nearly thirty years ago, Rudolf Jaenisch and Beatrice Mintz injected Simian virus 40 into the blastocoel cavity of preimplantation embryos, generating thereby the first transgenic animals (Jaenisch et al, PNAS1974). Subsequently, Jaenisch infected 2-4 cells stage embryos with a murine retrovirus and was able to report the successful transmission of the integrated viral DNA to the offspring (Jaenisch et al, 1976). These seminal works prompted different groups to replace viral genes with mammalian ones in order to express them ectopically in animals (Miller et al, 1997). These transgenes were present in all tissues analyzed and were transmitted to the offspring. However, the retrovirally delivered genes were not expressed in the transgenic animals. It was suggested that viral sequences in the long terminal repeats (LTR) could induce de novo methylation of host DNA and thereby interfere with gene expression during development (Jahner et al, Nature 1985). Thus, another technique was developed a few years later by injecting naked DNA directly into the pronucleus of a fertilized oocyte (Gordon et al, PNAS 1980). As most microinjected genes were expressed and were transmitted to progeny, it became the most widespread transgenic technology.

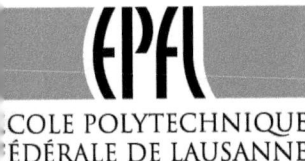

ÉCOLE POLYTECHNIQUE
FÉDÉRALE DE LAUSANNE

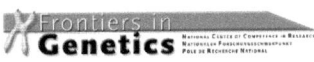

Acknowledgment

I would like to thanks for their good advices and critical readings Alexandra Liagre- Quazzola and Sonia Verp. Dr. F. Spitz for the pictures of embryos and N. Steiner and P. Herrera for their precious collaboration.

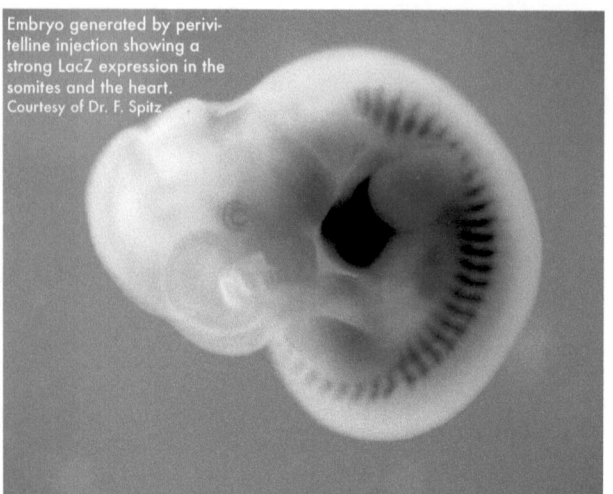

Embryo generated by perivitelline injection showing a strong LacZ expression in the somites and the heart.
Courtesy of Dr. F. Spitz

However, this technique was relatively inefficient, technically demanding and largely inapplicable to other species than the mouse. In 2002, the old idea of generating transgenic animal using a retrovirus was renewed thanks to the increasing knowledge in HIV biology. The successful development of lentiviral vector to mediate efficient in vivo delivery and long-term expression of a transgene combined with its relative escape of epigenetic silencing during development, made it become a valuable tool to generate transgenic animal (lois et al, Science 2002). Moreover, lentiviral transgenesis, due to its high efficacy combined with the relative ease to inject into the perivitelline space, became the most efficient method to generate transgenic livestock and poultry. The combination of lentiviral vectors with RNA interference was also used to silence the expression of specific genes in transgenic animals (Tiscornia Get al, PNAS 2003). In contrast to knock-out experiments using homologous recombination in embryonic stem cells (ES), lentiviral mediated transgenesis should allow gene targeting in species for which no ES cells are available. Furthermore, the development of a new drug-inducible system controlling the expression of pol II and pol III promoters opened the promising perspectives to regulate transgene expression or to induce the specific downregulation of a given gene (Szulc J et al, Nat Meth 2006).In the following protocol, I will describe the practical knowledge needed to generate transgenic mice.

Checklist

The experimental setting

The understage-illumination stereomicroscope
Stereomicroscopes Leica MZ7.5. We use this Leica to handle the embryos

Cold light motorized stereomicroscope
Again a Leica MZ7.5 but this time equipped with a discussion system that allows teaching. This stereomicroscope is used during the embryo transfer into the pseudopregnant mice. Noteworthy, the motorization of the focus is really convenient when both hand are used...

The station of injection
Leica ASTP (DIC contrast) with micromanipulators (Eppendorf NK2) and CellTram Air. Inject+matic. Anti-vibrations table (TMC), Holding:Vacutips sterile (Eppendorf, # 5175.108.000), loading tips: microloader (Eppendorf, # 5242.956.003) Excellent optic, the micromanipulator are easy to use. A must. The use of air instead of oil is an advantageous development in the holding setting. The anti-vibration tables offer a real comfort and speed up the whole procedure.

Microsurgical Instruments.
You will need one fine scissor, 2 watchmaker forceps n°5. Skin agrafes.
Silkman black USP 3/0 (Braun, # F1134043)
All our instruments were bought from Fine Science Tools

Reminder

Obtain the authorization from you legal authority to conduct animal experimentation

This could have been a chapter per se as the procedure is long and complicated, but it is beyond the scoop of this protocol and will vary from place to place, so just remember to contact early enough your local authority

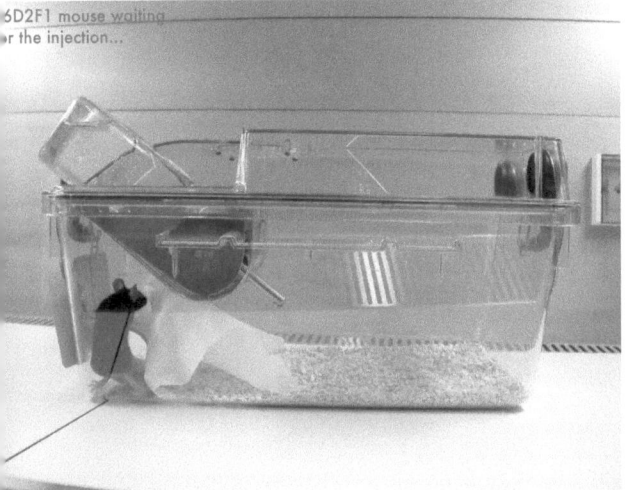

B6D2F1 mouse waiting for the injection...

Checklist

Hormone Injection

Monday 4pm
Pregnant Mare Serum (PMS)
10UI/mouse

Wednesday 2pm
Human Gonadotropin Hormone (hCG)
10UI/mouse

Wednesday 4pm
Mate the superovulated female with their male counterpart

Don't forget NMRI

Thursday 4pm

Mate NMRI with their vasectomized males (2 female/male)

Superovulation

This hybrid strains B6D2F1 derived from C57BL/6JxDBA2J are used as egg donor in our experiments. They are bought at 5 weeks of age from the Charles River company.

The superovulation starts three days before the collection of the embryo. Usually 5 B6D2F1 mice are injected intraperitonealy (IP) with 10U (100ul) of Pregnant Mare Serum (PMS) at 4 pm. Forty-six hours later, a second IP injection is made with 10U (100l) of Human Chorionic Gonadotropin (HCG). Following this injection, each female is individually mated with its male counterpart. Ideally, " fertile stud males" should be used in the prime of their life between 2 and 8 months and have 2-3 days of rest after the mating. In addition, a record of their performance should be maintained, as males having been mated successfully in the past (as indicated by a vaginal plug) are likely to do the same in the future. On average, we get 30-40 embryos per mouse

Vaginal plugs

The B6D2F1 female are checked for vaginal plug. To do so, each mouse is gently maintained by the tail. The female genitals are inspected visually for the presence of a crusty whitish plug called the vaginal plug that is the proof of a correct mating. This plug is the semen of the male that coagulate inside the vagina. Sometimes this plug can be difficult to visualize because it lies deeper into it. The use of a blunt instrument can help to gently open the mouse vaginal orifice and to feel the plug. If the plug is not seen, the mouse should not be used further and sacrifice, as we do not recycle superovulated mice. The plug check should be made in the morning as the

Chance for them to disappear increase with the delay between mating, which usually occur in the middle of the night and the plug check. For statistical purpose, each positive plug should be noted on the cage of the male.

Medium

The medium should be equilibrated in a C02 incubator at 37°C for min 30 min. One ml of "egg medium" (see appendix) should be added into two concave-shaped glass recipients called "saliere". In addition, two 3 cm dishes should be prepared with 4 droplets of 25ul of egg medium recovered by 2ml of mineral oil.

Isolating the eggs

B6D2F1 mice are anesthesized in a closed box containing isoflurane. As soon as the anesthesia is effective, the mice are killed by cervical dislocation. They are placed on their back. The fur is cleaned with ethanol 75%. The skin is ripped off and a longitudinal incision opens the peritoneum. The uteri are found by displacing the abdominal organs aside. A small dissection of the mesenterium will help to mobilize them. The ovaries are easily recognized at the tip of the uterus as a round redish structure recovered by the peri-ovarian fat pad. With the help of a forceps, the ligamentum ovari lying at the distal part of the ovary is gently grasped and an incision is made with fine scissors distally from the forceps. A second cut underneath the ovaries is made taking care not to touch the ampulla. Both the ovary and the ampulla are immediately put in the pre-warmed egg medium.

Then, under an understage-illumination stereomicroscope, the ampullas are opened by carefully tearing their wall using fine forceps, the embryos will then pop out. The ampulla is the bulged part of the oviduct and is normally easily visible. At this point, the embryos are still surrounded by numerous small cells forming the cumulus oophorus that the hyaluronidase will disaggregate. A few milligrammes (tip of a forceps) of hyaluronidase are added to the medium for 3 minutes at 37°C. The embryos are then washed in the second saliere. Afterwards, they are washed successively in the 3 droplets found in the petri dish. At this stage the embryos are counted and kept in the incubator until the injection of the lentivector. Injection chambers can now be prepared by adding two droplets of 5ul "egg medium" recovered with 750ul of 10S oil. They will be kept in the incubator at 37°C and 5%. CO_2.

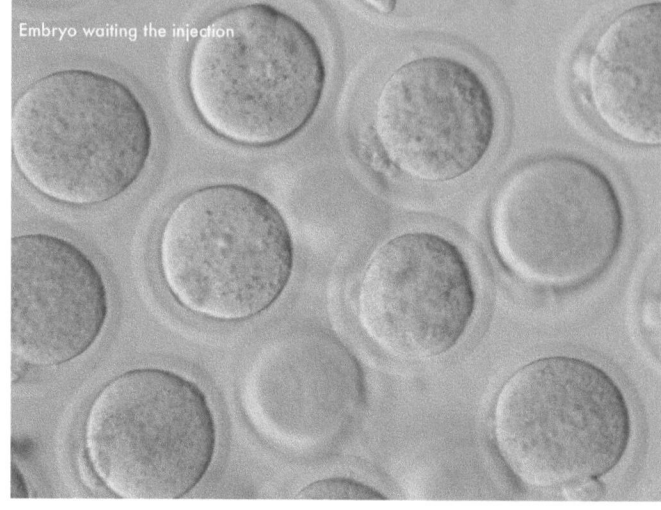

Embryo waiting the injection

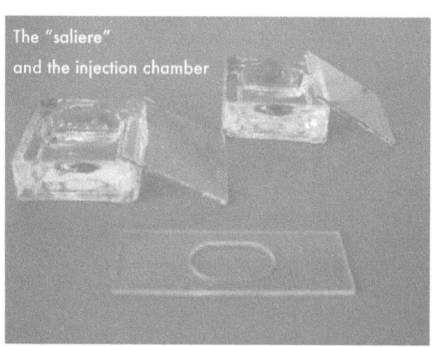

The "saliere" and the injection chamber

Checklist

Handling the embryos

Mouth pipette
To manipulate the embryos, we use a mouth pipette containing a fine capillary at its tip. This is very convenient but it requires some practice. Start with left over embryos

Washing step
It is important to wash rapidly the embryos after the 3 min hyaluronidase treatment. Moreover, try to take as minimum medium as possible while pipetting the embryos. Keep you embryos as often as possible in the incubator.

Ampulla
This is the bulged proximal part of the oviduct where all the embryos are collected. It is normally easily visible, but don't forget that sometime the mice do not respond to superovulation...

Timing
We start to isolate the embryos in the morning around 9am. The whole procedure should be finished just before noon which allows you to go for lunch and the embryos to recover

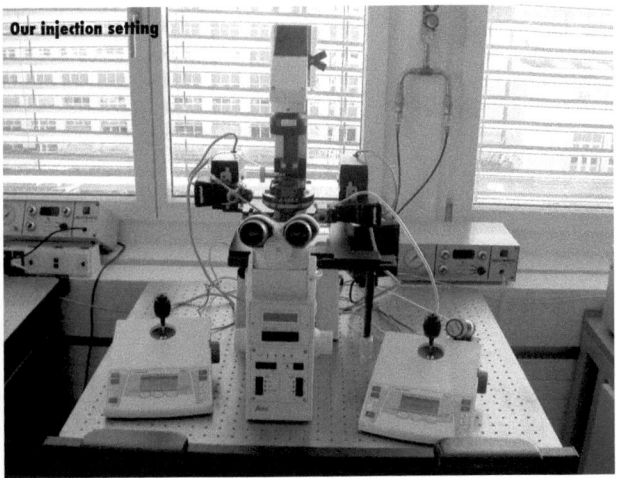

Our injection setting

The injection

The lentiviral vector preparation should be thawn on ice. Then, it is briefly vortexed and centrifuge in a bench centrifuge at fullspeed (13000rpm) for 5 min. The injection pipette is loaded with the lentiviral vector using a sequencing tip that is thin enough to be inserted into the capillary. A few microliters of vector is carefully loaded at the tip taking great care not to introduce air bubbles as the injection will then be impossible. The presence of air bubbles can be checked under a low magnification loupe. The holding and the injection pipette are positioned on their respective micromanipulator. Add 40 embryos per injection chamber and place it on the plate of the microscope. The micromanipulators are brought together and the microscope tour is placed back on its working position. The injectomatic is placed on "pressure" mode. Using the low magnification lens, the embryos should be visualized and focused at the center of the field. The shadow of the holding and the injection pipette should be seen on your left and right inside in order to allow their safe lowering under visual control (the injection pipette should always be injecting while passing through the oil layer). When they reached the bottom of the injection chamber, switch to high magnification lens and check if vector is released from the injection pipette. Place the holding and the injection pipette at the centre of the visual field. Embryos are underneath them and once injected, they are displaced in the upper part of the field. The lentiviral vector is injected into the perivitelline space next to the polar bodies. The amount of vector to be injected is difficult to calculate but as a rule of thumb, perform an injection of 2x 4-5 sec.
At the end, the embryo are washed successively in the 3 "egg medium"droplets found in the other 3cm petri dish and placed in the fourth one. Put 50 embryos per 50ul droplets max. An overnight incubation will allow the transfer of the divided embryos only.
At the end of the injection day, the foster mice NMRI are mated with vasectomized males (2 femelles per male).

Check list

Inject enough vectors

The vector
All vectors should have been correctly titered on HeLa cells and a cut-off limit of 5×10^8 HeLa transducing Unit/ml is the rule

Choice of embryos
Under high mag, an embryo should present two pronuclei, a nice round shape and often two polar bodies

Injecting pipette
To check if your pipette is injecting, find an air bubble at the bottom of the injection chamber. If the vector is delivered , the bubble should move away. If it is pluged, you can try to break its tip by hitting the the holding

Injecting the embryos
Try always to inject near the polar bodies as it will decrease the risk of breaching the plasma membrane. If it happens, then the embryo will dye.

After the injection
Mouth pipetting transduced embryos can be hazardous. To limitate such a risk, we interposed a 0.22um filter in the middle of the plastic tube of the mouth pipette. You can also use special pen-like pipette to handle your embryos

Warning
All the injection step should be performed in a state-of-the art P2 laboratory.

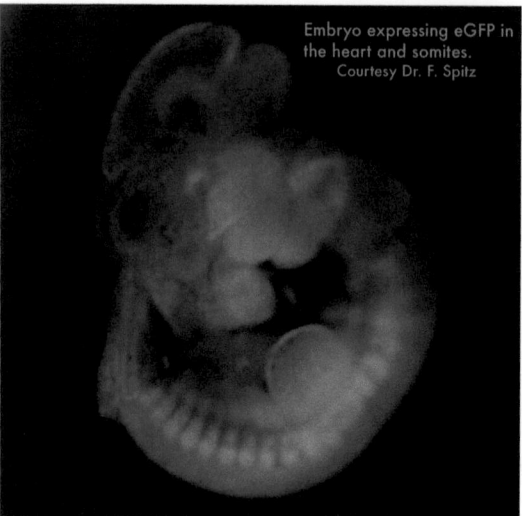

Embryo expressing eGFP in the heart and somites.
Courtesy Dr. F. Spitz

The transfer

The following day, vaginal plugs are checks. Usually 30 NMRI females are used to obtain between 3-5 successful matings. Next, an anaesthesia is performed by injecting IP 100ul of ketarum (cf Checklist) per 10 grammes of body weight. Protect the eye of the mouse with a drop of artificial tears in each eye. After ethanol disinfection, a small (1cm) incision is made longitudinally and caudally on the back, at the level of the last rib. The peri-ovarian fat is searched on both sides laterally and can be visualized through the peritoneum. Often a small peritoneal vessel can be observed in this area and is the landmark where the incision should be done. Pulling the ovarian fat pad with a fine forceps will bring the ovary out of the peritoneal cavity. When both ovaries have been pulled out, recover them with the overlaying skin, and collect 8 transduced embryos inside the capillary of a mouth pipette. Under a stereomicroscope, the ampulla is visualized as a dilatation of the oviduct. The sens of the ampulla should be determined and by gently grasping the undilated proximal part with a fine forceps, a small hole is made with a hypodermic needle. Without loosing eye contact, insert the embryo-containing capillary into this hole and inject them gently towards the ampulla. Ideally a small air bubble should be observed into it. At the end, the ovaries are put back in their primitive location and the peritoneum is sewed. After ethanol desinfection, the skin is clamped with agrafes. The mice are allowed to recover on a warmed plate, before being put back in their cage.

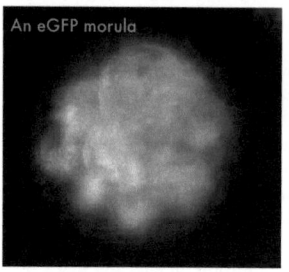

An eGFP morula

Check list

Take your time and don't drink coffee

Anesthezia

Ketarum is our anesthesic solution made of : Ketamin+Xylazin (see-suppl.) . It is convenient for brief anesthia. But as there are no antagonist, we usually inject 10% less of the required volume

Ovarian quest:look,look,look

Try first to visualize the peri-ovarian fat pad through the peritoneum. Usually, you will find an isolated small vessel in the proximity, cut nearby. If you don't succeed in pulling the ovary out, don't hesitate to increase the incision otherwise it will become haemorragic and you will also probably loose your grasp on the peri-ovarian fat pad

Loading the embryos

It is important to load the embryos in to the capillary with a minimal amount of medium. This will increase your transfer efficiency

Missed the Target? No second chance

Don't worry and keep cool! Try to pipette as many leftover embryo as you can around the ampulla and quickly wash them in medium. Change your capillary and try the other side. Don't come back to the first one

The end

Sometimes you will find difficult to put the ovary back into the peritoneal cavity. You can try to pull very laterally the peritoneum. It should help the ovary to slide back in place. A good tip is to add a few drops of PBS, it will then slide back easily

SYNOPSIS

y-3	**around 14h-16h** Start superovulation with the injection IP of 100ul (10U) of PMS/mouse Usually 5 mice will produce 150-200 oocytes
y-1	**around 12h-14h (46 hours after the first injection)** Injection IP of 100ul (10U) of HCG/mouse End of day, mate superovulated B6D2F1 One female per male
jection	**early in the morning control the vaginal plugs** Kill the superovulated mice Harvest oocytes using standard techniques. Leave the embryos in the saliere for 1-2 hours Perform the injection Wash the embryos 3 times Let them over night in the fourth droplet Mate the NMRI at the end of day 2-3 females/males Usually 3-5 plugs are reached when 30 NMRI are mated
y+1	**early in the morning check NMRI plugs** Check for the two cells stage embryos Transfer them into the ampulla of plugged NMRI Put the mice back into the conventional facilities

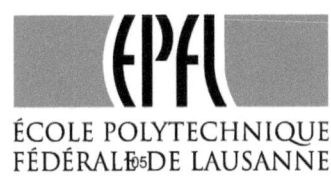

Annexe

Medium

Egg medium
-500ml MEM medium (Gibco, # 41090028)
-5ml Na PenStrep (10000UI/ml) (Invitrogen, # 15140122)
-1.33gr Na Lactate
-2gr BSA (Fluka, # A3311)
646ul Na Pyruvate (Fluka, # P4562)
Aliquot and store at -80°C

Oil
Mineral oil:
Store away from light (Fluka, # M5310)
Voltalef 10S (Verrerie de Carouge, # PR627-188)

Anesthesia

Ketarum
Ketamine+Xylazine
Rompun (20 mg/ml) + Ketalar (50 mg/ml)

Duration: 20-30min
Supplier:

Working solution
2.4ml Ketasol 50®
0.8ml Rompun®
6.8ml 0.9% NaCl
Take 0.1 ml/10g of mouse
Keep this solution for maximum 1 month

Artificial tears
Add one drop per eye
Supplier:

Hormones

Folligon (PMS): 1000UI
Dilute this powder in 10ml of 0.9% NaCl solution to obtain a final concentration of 10 U.I. Aliquot at 0.6ml into Eppendorf tubes, then stock the rest in the -80°C freezer. (Veterinaria, # 201.720)

Chorulon (hCG): 1500UI
Dilute the powder in 15ml of 0.9% NaCl solution to obtain a final concentration of 10 U.I. Aliquot and stock as described before (Veterinaria, # 201.718)

Choice of mouse strain

When setting up your transgenic facility, you will have to choose between the numerous mouse strains available. Grossly, there are two main stains: the inbred and the hybrid. The main advantage of an inbred strain such as the C57BL/6J is the genetic uniformity over time and space. Your mice are similar to those used ten years ago or in different lab around the world. Your control mouse will have the same genetic background as your experimental ones. Inbred strains eliminate the contribution of the genetic variability in the interpretation of the results. However, a totally inbred genome can produce detrimental phenotypic outcomes such as decreases fecundity, diminished resistance to pathogenes, etc..Therefore, you can prefer working in the vigor of an hybrid background, such as the B6D2F1 strain. Hybrid mice are generated by mating two inbred strains, in this example C57BL/6 with DBA. However, the mating of two hybrid will lead to a genotypically distinct offspring. To really be able to compare your transgenic animals in an hybrid background you will have to backcross it into a parental inbred strain.

M-O Sauvain

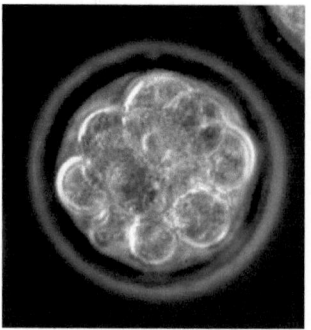

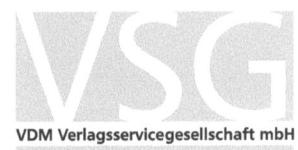

Die VDM Verlagsservicegesellschaft sucht für wissenschaftliche Verlage abgeschlossene und herausragende

Dissertationen, Habilitationen, Diplomarbeiten, Master Theses, Magisterarbeiten usw.

für die kostenlose Publikation als Fachbuch.

Sie verfügen über eine Arbeit, die hohen inhaltlichen und formalen Ansprüchen genügt, und haben Interesse an einer honorarvergüteten Publikation?

Dann senden Sie bitte erste Informationen über sich und Ihre Arbeit per Email an *info@vdm-vsg.de*.

Sie erhalten kurzfristig unser Feedback!

VDM Verlagsservicegesellschaft mbH
Dudweiler Landstr. 99　　　　　　　Telefon +49 681 3720 174
D - 66123 Saarbrücken　　　　　　　Fax　　+49 681 3720 1749
www.vdm-vsg.de

Die VDM Verlagsservicegesellschaft mbH vertritt

 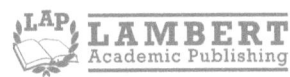 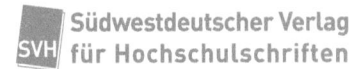

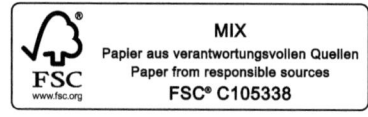

Printed by Books on Demand GmbH, Norderstedt / Germany